Fighting the Opioid Crisis with Communication

Xiaoxia Cao
Editor

Fighting the Opioid Crisis with Communication

Stigma, Treatment, Support, and Prevention

palgrave
macmillan

Editor
Xiaoxia Cao
University of Wisconsin–Milwaukee
Milwaukee, WI, USA

ISBN 978-3-032-31161-0 ISBN 978-3-032-31162-7 (eBook)
https://doi.org/10.1007/978-3-032-31162-7

This Palgrave Macmillan imprint is published by the registered company Springer Nature Switzerland AG.
The registered company address is: Gewerbestrasse 11, 6330 Cham, Switzerland

To those affected by the opioid crisis, and to those working to end it

Preface

When I received an invitation for serving as a guest editor of this book from Dr. Robin James, Editor for Media and Communications at Palgrave Macmillan, in February 2024, the annual opioid overdose deaths were declining. Although it offered some hope, the crisis was and still is far from over. Ending the crisis undoubtedly necessitates an integrated approach of which communication is a key component. For this reason, a group of communication scholars who have made meaningful contributions to our understanding of the role of communication in exacerbating and alleviating the crisis has come together in this edited volume to share their insights into how communication can help address this deadliest drug crisis in American history.

The chapters in this book demonstrate that effective communication strategies can be deployed to prevent opioid misuse, remove barriers to opioid use disorder (OUD) treatment and recovery, provide individuals with OUD the social support they need, and mobilize support for public health-oriented policies/interventions that help combat the crisis. Given the scope of this book, it should appeal to a wide range of audiences including, but not limited to, communication students and scholars with particular interests in interpersonal or mediated (health) communication, healthcare professionals particularly those prescribing opioid medications and interacting with patients with OUD, designers of communication campaigns/interventions, media content creators, and policy makers.

As a first-time book editor, I could not have completed this book project without the guidance, encouragement, and support of Dr. Robin James, who placed confidence in me, always provided the most straightforward answers to my questions, and made the entire project less daunting. My special thanks go to the contributors to this book. Some of them (e.g., Dr. Bagley and Dr. Wolfe) helped me assemble this excellent team of contributors by suggesting experts in the field who later became contributors; and others (e.g., Dr. Ledford) volunteered to change their writing plan to address reviewers' concerns. I was honored to work with each one of them and could not have asked for a better team!

University of Wisconsin–Milwaukee Xiaoxia Cao
Milwaukee, WI, USA

Contents

About the Editor and Contributors

About the Editor

Xiaoxia Cao (Ph.D., University of Pennsylvania) is an associate professor in the Department of Communication at the University of Wisconsin-Milwaukee. She is currently serving on the editorial board of Health Communication. Her research interests include health communication, media effects, persuasion, media psychology, and strategic communication.

About the Contributors

Braden H. Bagley (Ph.D., University of Southern Mississippi) is Assistant Professor of Strategic Communication at Southern Utah University. He specializes in several key areas of research, including health campaigns, crisis communication, and the interplay between communication and sports.

Jessica Beckham Houck (Ph.D., University of Southern Mississippi) is an assistant professor in the Department of Mass Media and Strategic Communication at the University of Tennessee at Martin. Her research focuses on health communication with particular interest in patient-provider interactions and methods to enhance patient outcomes.

Meghan N. Breckling (Doctor of Pharmacy, University of Arkansas for Medical Sciences [UAMS]) is an assistant professor at UAMS, College of Pharmacy in the Department of Pharmacy Practice, Center for Implementation Research. Her current research interests include improving healthcare provider education on opioid-related topics.

Hayden V. Coombs (Ph.D., Northcentral University) is Assistant Professor of Sports Communication at Southern Utah University. His research areas include institutional inequities in collegiate athletics and sports management.

Jacqueline N. Gunning (M.A., University of Nebraska–Lincoln) is a doctoral student studying interpersonal and health communication in the Department of Communication at the University of Connecticut. Her research focuses on how individuals approach difficult conversations about health and how those conversations shape their health behaviors and outcomes.

Virgil L. Hayes Jr. (Ph.D., University of Missouri) is an assistant teaching professor in the College of Health Sciences at the University of Missouri. His work focuses on scale design, framing effects, and advancing theorizing in areas of stigma communication.

Elizabeth A. Hintz (Ph.D., University of South Florida) is an assistant professor in the Department of Communication at the University of Connecticut. Her research examines how people managing complex, stigmatized, and poorly understood health conditions navigate challenging conversations with partners, family members, and clinicians.

Övgü Kaynak (Ph.D., Temple University) is Associate Professor of Psychology at Penn State Harrisburg. Her research lies in the intersection of psychology and public health and focuses on building motivation, resiliency, and coping skills to provide people with expanded opportunities for living safe and productive lives.

Nathan E. Kruis (Ph.D., Indiana University of Pennsylvania) is Associate Professor of Criminal Justice at Penn State Altoona and research associate at the Douglas W. Pollock Center for Addiction Outreach and Research. His research interests include policing, criminological theory, stigma, substance use, and criminal justice pedagogy.

Victoria A. Ledford (Ph.D., University of Maryland) is Assistant Professor of Health Communication at Auburn University. She conducts research on how public stigma is communicated and what strategies can counter stigma, particularly in the opioid context.

Leah R. Tobey-Moore (Doctor of Physical Therapy, University of Central Arkansas) is an assistant professor in the Center for Health Services Research in the Department of Psychiatry with a secondary appointment in the Department of Geriatrics at the University of Arkansas for Medical Sciences (UAMS). She is the Lead Trainer for the SAMHSA-funded Arkansas Naloxone Education Training (ANET) Program.

Lili R. Romann (M.A., University of Connecticut) is a doctoral student at the University of Connecticut. Her research lies in the nexus of interpersonal health and computer-mediated communication with an emphasis on (stigmatized) health experiences and health information-seeking processes.

Christopher R. Whipple (Ph.D., DePaul University) is Associate Professor of Psychology at Penn State Harrisburg. His current research utilizes basic and applied research to develop, implement, and evaluate community-based interventions and to inform intervention development and targets.

Brooke H. Wolfe (Ph.D., University of Washington) is currently the Dean's Postdoctoral Fellow in the Department of Communication at Michigan State University. Her research focuses on the communication of individuals historically marginalized, and underrepresented, within interpersonal, family, and health contexts.

List of Figures

List of Tables

CHAPTER 1

Fighting the Opioid Crisis with Communication: Stigma, Treatment, Support, and Prevention

Xiaoxia Cao

1.1 Introduction

The American opioid crisis has devastating public health, economic, and social consequences. A 2024 national survey found that more than 8 million Americans aged 12 or older misused opioids in the past year, which includes prescription opioids (7.57 million), heroin (0.56 million), and illegally made fentanyl (0.67 million; Substance Abuse and Mental Health Administration 2025). Although drug overdose deaths dropped by 27% in 2024 compared with 2023, there were still more than 80,000 Americans losing their lives to drug overdoses in 2024 (Anderer 2025), and the vast majority of the deaths (i.e., 73%) involved at least one opioid (U.S. Centers for Disease Control and Prevention 2025). The opioid crisis has cost Americans more than $1 trillion a year since 2017 (Kuehn 2021). For example, illicit opioids, primarily fentanyl, alone cost taxpayers an

X. Cao (✉)
Department of Communication, University of Wisconsin-Milwaukee,
Milwaukee, WI, USA
e-mail: xcao@uwm.edu

X. Cao (ed.), *Fighting the Opioid Crisis with Communication*,
https://doi.org/10.1007/978-3-032-31162-7_1

estimated $2.7 trillion in 2023, including reduced labor productivity, hike in healthcare cost, and increase in crime-related expenses (The White House 2025).

In addition, the opioid crisis has strained social relationships, destroyed families, ruined childhood, and fueled crime (Brundage et al. 2019). For example, an estimated 2 million children in the U.S. were directly impacted by the crisis in 2017. These children had been living with a parent with opioid use disorder (OUD), lost a parent to an opioid-related death, had a parent imprisoned due to opioids and/or been removed from their home as the result of opioid-related issues. There is also evidence linking the rise of opioid-related crime to the increase of opioid misuse (indicated by opioid-related ER visits, hospitalization and overdose mortality; Chen et al. 2022).

This chapter begins with a review of the development of the current opioid crisis in the U.S. along with a discussion of its contributing factors, with an emphasis on the role of communication in facilitating the development. After this, the chapter lays out how communication can be part of the solution to the crisis and how each chapter in this volume contributes to our understanding of the role of communication in combating the crisis.

1.2 The American Opioid Crisis and Contributing Factors

The current American opioid crisis is not the first in history (Patel and Rushefsky 2022). The first one started in the 1860s and lasted until the 1920s, during which opioid medications such as morphine and heroin (diacetylmorphine) were widely used to treat physical and mental pain. Their use provoked a hunger for increased doses of the medications, leading to addiction. To address the problem, a law was passed in 1909 to prohibit the possession, distribution, or sale of opium for non-medical use (Spitz 2020), which was followed by the Harrison Narcotics Tax Act of 1914. The Act essentially sanctioned the use of narcotics for most medical conditions. Violators could face up to more than $50,000 in fines in modern U.S. dollars and up to 5 years in prison. The enactment of these laws began a period of opiophobia between the 1920s and 1970s, when severe pain was undertreated even among the terminally ill.

In the 1970s, opinions about opioid medications among healthcare professionals started to budge following an article published by *the Annals of Internal Medicine* in 1973 (Spitz 2020, 83). In the article, two doctors, Richard Marks and Edward Sachar, highlighted the needless suffering of medical patients due to the underutilization of narcotics. They argued that physicians often underestimated effective doses of opioid painkillers and overestimated the addiction risk of the medical use of opioids. The article reinvigorated the discussion surrounding the use of opioids for pain management. Nonetheless, opioid painkillers were still prescribed primarily for acute pain resulting from injury or surgery or severe pain associated with cancer or terminal illnesses throughout the 1970s. Physicians were reluctant to prescribe opioids for other conditions because of a concern for addiction and the lack of evidence supporting wider prescribing practices. However, this practice would soon be challenged.

In 1980, *the New England Journal of Medicine* published a one-paragraph letter to the editor in which Jane Porter and Hershel Jick questioned the practice of using opioids mainly for treating acute pain based on their retrospective review of the medical records of 11,882 patients who had received at least one opioid painkiller during inpatient care between 1970 and 1979 (Rummans et al. 2018, 345). The review showed that only 4 of the over 11 thousand patients became addicted to opioids. This one-paragraph letter, however, failed to provide information necessary for evaluating the validity of its conclusion, such as the dose and the length of the opioid treatment received by the patients. Nonetheless, the letter was referenced over 600 times to support the use of opioids to treat chronic pain. Its wide publicity started to ease the concern for addiction associated with opioid medications. Then, in the textbook titled *Narcotic Analgesics in Anesthesiology*, published in 1982, Arther Taub claimed that the continuation of opioid therapy in patients with non-cancer pain would not increase the risk of substance abuse or psychological dependence, which compelled some physicians, professional organizations, and even the World Health Organization (WHO) to start advocating for expanding the use of opioids for pain control.

Convinced that America was "a nation awash in chronic pain that could only be relieved if only the medical profession would overcome its prejudice" and fear toward opioids, a group of medical professionals started to aggressively promote a series of claims they said were rooted in scientific evidence (McGreal 2018). One of the claims was that it was not possible for patients genuinely experiencing pain to become addicted to opioids because "the pain neutralized the euphoria caused by the narcotic" and the drug dependence displayed by patients on opioid painkillers was "pseudo-addiction."

In 1986, two advocates for the expansion of opioid treatment, Russell Portenoy and Kathleen Foley, published their study of 38 patients with chronic non-cancer pain who received ongoing opioid treatment (Spitz 2020, 86). Their data showed that out of the 38 patients, only two with a history of substance abuse misused the drugs. Based on this observation, the two researchers concluded that addiction to opioid painkillers could be avoided if doctors screened patients for their medical history. Later, Portenoy toured the country, touting that opioids were a "gift from nature" and promoting their access was a moral obligation (McGreal 2018). He even claimed that opioids "can be used for a long time, with few side-effects, and that addiction and abuse are not a problem." Years later, when the opioid crisis was in its full-blown, Portenoy admitted that his claims were not well-founded.

Also in 1986, the WHO released comprehensive guidelines to expand cancer pain management (Spitz 2020, 85). The guidelines supported the notion that freedom of pain (not just severe pain), especially among the terminally ill, is a human right. They advised healthcare providers to take complaints of pain from patients seriously and treat them following an analgesic ladder that specified a standardized way of escalating pain treatment among cancer patients. The implementation of the guidelines was a huge success. Patients treated under the guidelines reported little change in functioning, and retrospective reviews of patient data found no link between the use of opioid painkillers and addiction. These observations combined with the effectiveness of opioid therapy in alleviating cancer pain and the belief that it is a human right to be pain-free led to the beginning of a slow but steady increase in the use of opioids for treating anyone experiencing pain in the late 1980s. From 1990 to 1995, opioid prescriptions increased by 2 to 3 million each year (Rummans et al. 2018, 346).

This increase was accelerated by several major developments in the mid-1990s and early 2000s that set in motion the deadliest drug crisis in American history. In 1995, the U.S. Food and Drug Administration (FDA) approved OxyContin (oxycodone extended-release), manufactured by Purdue Pharma, for the long-term treatment of moderate-to-severe pain, cancer-related or not, that lasts for more than a few days (Woodcock 2013). After receiving the green light from the FDA, Purdue Pharma started its aggressive OxyContin marketing campaigns (Rummans et al. 2018, 346). As a result, annual prescriptions of OxyContin for pain management increased from 670,000 to 6.2 million between 1997 and 2002 (Rummans et al. 2018, 346), making it the leading opioid medication on the market (Brown and Morgan 2019, 3).

Not coincidentally, the year after OxyContin received FDA approval, the now-defunct American Pain Society (APS), an organization partly funded by pharmaceutical companies, started to push the notion of pain as the "fifth vital sign" (McGreal 2018). The president of the society, James Campbell, told members of the society that "if pain were assessed with the same zeal as other vital signs are, it would have a much better chance of being treated properly. We need to train doctors and nurses to treat pain as a vital sign." In the same year, the American Academy of Pain Medicine (AAPM) and the APS issued a joint statement, acknowledging the role of opioids in treating chronic non-cancer pain (Rummans et al. 2018, 345). At the same time, several studies were published that documented the prevalence of untreated pain among various populations (e.g., patients with cancer, AIDS, or hospitalized in the Intensive Care Units; Rummans et al. 2018, 346). Subsequently, many states passed the Intractable Pain Acts, eliminating sanctions for physicians who prescribed opioids for long-term use and, therefore, removing a major hurdle to the massive prescription of opioids.

In 2001, new guidelines for monitoring and treating pain were issued by the Joint Commission, an organization that sets the standards and monitors the quality of patient care provided by hospitals and medical centers (Rummans et al. 2018, 347). The new guidelines emphasized the need for systematic assessments of pain experienced by inpatients along with four other vital signs (i.e., pulse, blood pressure, temperature and respiration). Pain, thus, officially became the fifth vital sign. Afterward, the Deficit Reduction Act of 2005 required hospitals to participate in the Hospital Consumer Assessment of Healthcare Providers and Systems Survey (HCAHPSS). Three out of the twenty-five questions on the patient satisfaction survey were related to pain management. Participation in the survey was directly linked to the annual payment received by hospitals via the Inpatient Prospective Payment System. Later, the results of the survey were used to decide which hospitals would receive financial rewards for providing high-quality care. Given that pain management greatly influenced the results of the patient satisfaction survey, doctors felt pressured to prescribe more opioid pain medication.

After three decades in the making, the opioid crisis was in full swing. Between 2000 and 2010, prescription opioid use quadrupled (Spitz 2020,

86). Opioid prescription per capita peaked between 2010 and 2012 when 81 out of every 100 Americans had an opioid prescription. In 2012 alone, Americans used 165,525 kilograms of opioids, relative to 46,946 kilograms in 2000, despite no change in the amount of pain experienced during that time. This dramatic increase in the use of prescription opioids for pain relief led to a surge in opioid dependence and overdose deaths in the U.S. Between 2000 and 2010, the rate of overdose deaths involving at least one opioid more than doubled from 2.9 to 6.8 per 100,000 Americans (Duff et al. 2022). This initial rise of opioid-related deaths, caused mainly by prescription opioids, is widely considered the first wave of the opioid crisis.

In the 2010s, increased concern about opioid dependence and overdose led to a series of changes that reduced opioid prescriptions (Brown and Morgan 2019, 4). In 2010, Purdue Pharma reformulated OxyContin to make it more difficult to crush or dissolve for illicit use. Prescribing guidelines, taking into consideration the risks associated with prescription opioids, were issued. Electronic prescription drug monitoring programs (PDMPs) were adopted by more states, which helped reduce inappropriate opioid prescribing by physicians and doctor shopping by patients. Subsequently, opioid prescription rates fell by 40% between 2011 and the late 2010s (Aitken 2020, 2).

While the supply of prescription opioids became more restricted, heroin became increasingly available at a record-low price (Duff et al. 2022, 1). As a result, people who misused prescription opioids turned to heroin to satisfy their craving for opioids. Subsequently, the use of heroin in the U.S. increased sharply between 2010 and 2015 (Brown and Morgan 2019, 4), which led to a nearly fivefold increase in heroin-involved overdose deaths from 1.0 to 5.9 per 100,000 people between 2010 and 2016 (Duff et al. 2022, 1). In 2015, heroin surpassed prescription opioids, becoming the leading cause of overdose deaths involving an opioid. The rise of heroin overdose deaths is often referred to as the second wave of the opioid crisis.

Fentanyl, a type of very potent synthetic opioid, started to emerge in the U.S. around 2013 (Brown and Morgan 2019, 5). In 2016, fentanyl became the leading cause of drug overdose deaths in the U.S., accounting for 29% of such deaths (Brown and Morgan 2019, 6). Between 2015 and 2020, the rate of opioid-involved drug overdose deaths—mainly caused by fentanyl—doubled from 10.4 to 21.4 per 100, 000 Americans. The rise of opioid overdose deaths driven by fentanyl is often considered the third wave of the opioid crisis (Duff et al. 2022, 1).

Since 2019, the U.S. has been experiencing the fourth wave of the opioid crisis, characterized by drug overdose deaths driven by polysubstance misuse that involves fentanyl and stimulants such as methamphetamine and cocaine (Friedman and Shover 2023, 2477). The percentage of overdose deaths involving a combination of fentanyl and stimulants increased from 0.6% in 2010 to 32.3% in 2021, with the sharpest rise starting in 2015. By 2023, more than 800,000 Americans had died from a drug overdose involving at least one opioid since 1999 (U.S. Centers for Disease Control and Prevention 2025), making the current opioid crisis the deadliest drug crisis in American history.

Causes of the opioid crisis are many (Blanco et al. 2020). Overprescribing opioid pain medications is undoubtedly a significant contributor. This overreliance on opioids for pain management can be partly attributed to various policies. For example, government agencies have issued misguided policies on using opioids for pain management (Spitz 2020, 86). Health insurance policies usually restrict the reimbursement of more costly but less addictive pain therapy (Rummans et al. 2018, 347). Of course, as aforementioned, the easy accessibility of illicit opioids also fuels the crisis (Duff et al. 2022). In addition, many believe that the crisis has its root in social and economic upheaval characterized by "the lack of economic opportunity, poor working conditions, and eroded social capital in depressed communities, accompanied by hopelessness and despair" (Dasgupta et al. 2018, 184). Fatal drug overdoses, therefore—along with alcohol-related disease and suicide—are considered "diseases of despair" (Dasgupta et al. 2018, 183). To be specific, lower-middle-class white Americans have been experiencing reduced economic opportunities and declined living standards in the post-industrial era (Brown and Morgan 2019, 6). The social and psychological stress resulting from economic hardship has been linked to physical pain (e.g., lower back pain) that intensifies the (mis)use of opioids (Dasgupta et al. 2018, 184).

That said, the role of communication in facilitating the development of the opioid crisis is undeniable. The development can be partly attributed to the misunderstanding of the dangers of opioids as a pain management tool among healthcare professionals, government officials, and the public that was largely induced and perpetuated by misleading communication from researchers, professional organizations, and pharmaceutical companies. For example, the publication of questionable studies that downplayed the addictive nature of opioid pain medications—the most prominent of which were that by Jane Porter and Hershel Jick published in 1980 and the one by Russell Portenoy and Kathleen Foley published in 1986 (Rummans et al. 2018, 345; Spitz 2020, 86)—changed the perceptions of risks associated with using opioids to manage non-cancer chronic pain among healthcare professionals, even though the findings of these studies are inconsistent with the results of more rigorous research. To make matters worse, these questionable studies were widely cited by some physicians and professional organizations (e.g., APS) to support their aggressive campaigns for expanding the use of opioid therapy (Spitz 2020).

The marketing campaigns of pharmaceutical companies also propelled the development of the opioid crisis. For example, Purdue Pharma created and distributed more than 15,000 copies of the video titled "I got my life back" to physician offices. In the video, six patients who were prescribed OxyContin for chronic non-cancer pain shared their positive experiences with the medication. The promotional video not only encouraged physicians to use the product for ongoing treatment of chronic pain but also assured them that the drug was free of side effects. In addition, the company funded pro-opioid-use educational programs and promoted research in favor of opioid use (Brown and Morgan 2019, 4). To further increase the demand for OxyContin, Purdue Pharma used TV commercials to target consumers with chronic pain including 70 million Americans with lower back pain (Leibovici 2023, 128). The marketing efforts of pharmaceutical companies are linked directly to opioid misuse and related deaths. For example, research has shown that states with higher exposure to OxyContin introduction campaigns had higher annual increases in overdose deaths since 1996 (Alpert et al. 2022). While the misleading marketing campaigns by pharmaceutical companies were attempting to put as many Americans as possible on opioid therapy, not enough effort was made by governments and health organizations to educate the public and healthcare professionals about the dangers of opioid medications, which was also responsible for the development of the opioid crisis (Spitz 2020).

In addition to influencing risk perceptions associated with opioid medications and shaping the pain management practices of healthcare professionals, communication has contributed to the exacerbation of the opioid crisis by creating barriers to OUD treatment and recovery. A survey conducted in 2022 found that only 25% of people with OUD received medications proven to substantially reduce opioid-related mortality (i.e., buprenorphine and methadone), 30% received treatment without the medications, and 45% did not receive any treatment (Dowell et al. 2024). Moreover, people with OUD often have difficulty gaining the social support necessary for recovery and reintegration into society (Krendl and Perry 2023; Park et al. 2023).

One important contributing factor to the low treatment rate and the lack of social support is stigma toward individuals with OUD (Hammarlund et al. 2018), defined as "a mark of shame, disgrace or disapproval which results in an individual being rejected, discriminated against, and excluded from participating in a number of different areas of society" (World Health Organization 2001, 32). The stigma perpetuated by interpersonal and mediated communication, as discussed in Chaps. 2, 3, 4 and 5 of this edited volume, is linked to poor mental and physical health (Ahern et al. 2007), delays in seeking treatment, higher treatment withdrawal (Perry et al. 2020; Tsai et al. 2019), withholding information necessary for receiving care and support (Krendl and Perry 2023), and reluctance to carry potential life-saving medicine (e.g., Naloxone; Bennett et al., 2020) among people with drug use disorder. The stigma is also associated with increased support for discriminatory policies that make it difficult for people with OUD to reintegrate into society (Kennedy-Hendricks et al. 2017). Moreover, the stigma undermines support for public health-focused policies that facilitate OUD treatment and recovery. Hence, it is fair to say that communication fueled the growth of the opioid crisis by creating an opinion climate that was conducive to the expansion of opioid use and, at the same time, hindered the treatment and recovery of individuals with OUD.

1.3 Fighting the Opioid Crisis with Communication

To combat the opioid crisis, it necessitates to promote OUD recovery and prevention via an integrated approach, in which communication plays an essential role. To improve the well-being of chronic pain patients who benefit from opioid therapy and those with OUD, it is important to understand how chronic pain (patients), people with OUD, OUD medications, and harm reduction measures (e.g., carrying Narcan and syringe exchange programs) are being stigmatized via interpersonal and mediated communication and what language, portrayals, and message frames can be adopted to reverse the stigmatization, promote OUD recovery, and rally support for harm reduction measures. These are the focus of Part I of this book.

In Chapter 2, Dr. Kaynak and her colleagues review the current literature on stigma toward individuals with OUD, language used to stigmatize people with OUD, their behavior, OUD treatment, as well as the consequences of the stigmatization. The chapter ends with evidence-based recommendations for replacing stigmatizing language with person-first, non-stigmatizing language to bring about positive social changes. In Chap. 3, Dr. Ledford provides a comprehensive review of research into the portrayals of people with OUD by news, entertainment, and social media. The review analyzes the media portrayals via the lens of stigma communication and sheds light on stigmatizing media depictions of people with OUD. The chapter concludes with recommendations for creating more de-stigmatizing and humanizing portrayals of people with OUD.

Chapter 4 focuses on framing used to communicate about people with OUD, harm reduction measures, and drug policies. In the chapter, Dr. Hayes reviews studies investigating the impacts of message framing on causal attribution of OUD, stigma toward individuals with OUD, support for treatment and harm reduction programs, and opinions toward punitive or public health-oriented policy approaches to combating the opioid crisis. The chapter ends with a detailed discussion of how future framing-effects research can continue improving our understanding of the attitudinal, behavioral, and policy implications of various ways of framing OUD, OUD-related treatment, programs, and policies. In Chap. 5, Dr. Hintz and her associates report a content analysis of newspaper coverage of chronic pain (patient) in the context of the opioid crisis between 2012 and 2022. The analysis revealed the dominant frames, prominent characters, and significant events present in the coverage, which improves our understanding of the portrayals of chronic pain (patients) by the news media and sheds light on the potential harm these portrayals may cause to people with chronic pain. The chapter concludes with suggestions for improving media coverage of chronic pain (patients) to avoid harming this population while addressing the issues of opioid overprescription and misuse. Together, the four chapters in the first section of this book not only highlight the problematic practices used to communicate about OUD, individuals with OUD, OUD treatment, harm reduction measures, policy interventions, and chronic pain (patients) but also provide guidance for improving communication practices in order to destigmatize people with OUD and OUD treatment, increase support for harm reduction measures and public health-oriented policies, and enhance the well-being of those suffering from OUD and/or chronic pain.

As one ounce of prevention is worth a pound of cure, prevention must be a crucial part of the plan for fighting the opioid crisis. Thus, Part II of this book reveals how communication can be deployed to prevent opioid misuse. In Chap. 6, Dr. Bagley and Dr. Coombs outline a host of messaging strategies—rooted in the Extended Parallel Process Model (EPPM) and the Health Belief Model (HBM)—that can be used by campaign designers to influence the audience's attitudes and behaviors and prevent opioid misuse. These strategies include, but are not limited to, highlighting the potential harm that misusing opioids may cause and improving self, response, and system efficacy through communicating tangible resources and social support that are available. Complementing the strategies detailed in Chap. 6, the study reported in Chap. 7 demonstrates how the reference focus of anti-prescription opioid messages may influence the effectiveness of such messages. Using a two-stage online experiment with two between-subjects conditions, the study tested the immediate and delayed impacts of the reference focus (self vs. self-other) of anti-prescription opioid risk narratives on the effectiveness of the narratives as well as the mediating roles of fear and anticipated guilt. Its findings suggest that self-focused risk narratives and messages arousing anticipated guilt may be effective in bringing about attitudinal and behavioral changes that reduce the likelihood of opioid misuse.

Unlike Chaps. 6 and 7, which focus on preventing opioid misuse through influencing the attitudes and behaviors of the public, Chap. 8 explores how to prevent opioid misuse by deploying communication strategies to improve the prescribing practices of healthcare professionals. In the chapter, Dr. Breckling and Dr. Tobey-Moore reveal how academic detailing (AD), a one-on-one or small-group outreach education strategy, can help healthcare professionals better implement evidence-based safer opioid prescribing practices, which include safer initiation and dosing, follow-up, and harm reduction. The chapter ends with recommendations for improving AD communication strategies and a discussion of possible future research that can help further optimize the impact of AD in the context of the opioid crisis. Thus, the three chapters in Part II of the book showcase how communication can be used to influence the knowledge, attitudes, and behavior of the public and healthcare professionals and prevent opioid misuse.

To end the opioid crisis, it is important to help people with OUD to recover. Hence, the two chapters in Part III of this book examine how communication can be used to facilitate treatment and recovery. In Chap. 9, Dr. Houck explores OUD treatment strategies via the lens of the ecological model. The chapter emphasizes the importance of using patient-centered communication and patient navigation to address multi-level barriers that shape the outcome of OUD treatment. Finally, in Chap. 10, Dr. Wolfe and Dr. Hintz use the Communication Theory of Resilience to evaluate a popular peer support program that helps individuals suffering from substance use disorders, including OUD, enter and maintain recovery. The chapter ends with recommendations for improving the program and, therefore, the peer support available to individuals with OUD.

Collectively, the chapters in this book demonstrate that communication should and must be part of the solution to the opioid crisis because communication helps prevent opioid misuse by influencing the knowledge, attitudes, and behaviors of the public and health professionals; remove barriers to OUD treatment and recovery; mobilize public support for harm reduction and public health approach to addressing the crisis; and provide individuals with OUD the social support they desperately need for recovery. Understanding the role of communication in combating the opioid crisis and adopting the recommendations proposed in this book by media content producers, the public, healthcare professionals, designers of communication interventions, and policy makers will undoubtedly bring us a step closer to ending this deadliest drug crisis in American history.

References

Anderer, Samantha. 2025. US Drug Overdose Deaths Dropped Nearly 27% Last Year. *JAMA* 334 (2): 107. https://doi.org/10.1001/jama.2025.7795.

Ahern, Jennifer, Jennifer Stuber, and Sandro Galea. 2007. Stigma, Discrimination and the Health of Illicit Drug Users. *Drug and Alcohol Dependence* 88 (2–3): 188–196. https://doi.org/10.1016/j.drugalcdep.2006.10.014.

Aitken, Murray. 2020. *Prescription Opioid Trends in the United States: Measuring and Understanding Progress in the Opioid Crisis.* IQVIA Institute for Human Data Science. https://www.iqvia.com/-/media/iqvia/pdfs/institute-reports/prescription-opioid-trends-in-the-united-states/iqi-prescription-opioid-trends-in-the-us-1220-forweb.pdf.

Alpert, Abby, William N. Evans, Ethan M. J. Lieber, and David Powell. 2022. Origins of the Opioid Crisis and Its Enduring Impacts. *The Quarterly Journal of Economics* 137 (2): 1139–1179. https://doi.org/10.1093/qje/qjab043.

Bennett, Alex S., Robert Freeman, Don C. Des Jarlais, and Ian David Aronson. 2020. Reasons People Who Use Opioids Do Not Accept or Carry No-Cost Naloxone: Qualitative Interview Study. *JMIR Formative Research* 4 (12): e22411. https://doi.org/10.2196/22411.

Blanco, Carlos, Tisha R. A. Wiley, Jacqueline J. Lloyd, Marsha F. Lopez, and Nora D. Volkow. 2020. America's Opioid Crisis: The Need for an Integrated Public Health Approach. *Translational Psychiatry* 10 (1): 167. https://doi.org/10.1038/s41398-020-0847-1.

Brown, Rick, and Anthony Morgan. 2019. The Opioid Epidemic in North America: Implications for Australia. *Trends and Issues in Crime and Criminal Justice 578*:1–15.

Brundage, Suzanne C., Adam Fifield, and Lee Patridge. 2019. The Ripple Effect: National and State Estimates of the U.S. Opioid Epidemic's Impact on Children. United Hospital Fund. https://media.uhfnyc.org/filer_public/6e/80/6e80760f-579-46a3-998d-1aa816ab06f6/uhf_ripple_effect_national_and_state_estimates_chartbook.pdf.

Chen, Qiushi, Glenn Sterner, Joel Segel, and Zixuan Feng. 2022. Trends in Opioid-Related Crime Incidents and Comparison with Opioid Overdose Outcomes in the United States. *International Journal of Drug Policy* 101:103555. https://doi.org/10.1016/j.drugpo.2021.103555.

Dasgupta, Nabarun, Leo Beletsky, and Daniel Ciccarone. 2018. Opioid Crisis: No Easy Fix to Its Social and Economic Determinants. *American Journal of Public Health* 108 (2): 182–186. https://doi.org/10.2105/AJPH.2017.304187.

Dowell, Deborah, Samantha Brown, Shiromani Gyawali, et al. 2024. Treatment for Opioid Use Disorder: Population Estimates—United States, 2022. *MMWR. Morbidity and Mortality Weekly Report* 73 (25): 567–574. https://doi.org/10.15585/mmwr.mm7325a1.

Duff, Johnathan H., Joanna R. Lampe, Liana W. Rosen, and Wen W. Shen. 2022. *The Opioid Crisis in the United States: A Brief History.* Congressional Research Service. https://www.congress.gov/crs-product/IF12260.

Friedman, Joseph, and Chelsea L. Shover. 2023. Charting the Fourth Wave: Geographic, Temporal, Race/Ethnicity and Demographic Trends in Polysubstance Fentanyl Overdose Deaths in the United States, 2010–2021. *Addiction* 118 (12): 2477–2485. https://doi.org/10.1111/add.16318.

Hammarlund, Rebecca A., Kathleen A. Crapanzano, Lauren Luce, Lauren A. Mulligan, and Kathleen M. Ward. 2018. Review of the Effects of Self-Stigma and Perceived Social Stigma on the Treatment-Seeking Decisions of Individuals with Drug- and Alcohol-Use Disorders. *Substance Abuse and Rehabilitation* 9:115–136. https://doi.org/10.2147/SAR.S183256.

Kennedy-Hendricks, Alene, Colleen L. Barry, Sarah E. Gollust, Margaret E. Ensminger, Margaret S. Chisolm, and Emma E. McGinty. 2017. Social Stigma toward Persons with Prescription Opioid Use Disorder: Associations with Public Support for Punitive and Public Health–Oriented Policies. *Psychiatric Services* 68 (5): 462–469. https://doi.org/10.1176/appi.ps.201600056.

Krendl, Anne C., and Brea L. Perry. 2023. Stigma Toward Substance Dependence: Causes, Consequences, and Potential Interventions. *Psychological Science in the Public Interest*24(2):90–126.https://doi.org/10.1177/15291006231198193.

Kuehn, Bridget M. 2021. Massive Costs of the US Opioid Epidemic in Lives and Dollars. *JAMA* 325 (20): 2040. https://doi.org/10.1001/jama.2021.7464.

McGreal, Chris. 2018. The Making of an Opioid Epidemic: When High Doses of Painkillers Led to Widspread Addiction, It Was Called One of the Biggest Mistakes in Modern Medicine. But This Was No Accident. The Guardian, November 8. https://www.theguardian.com/news/2018/nov/08/the-making-of-an-opioid-epidemic.

Leibovici, Bertrand L. 2023. The American Opioid Crisis and the Future of Drug Policies. *International Journal on Criminology* 10 (1): 125–134.

Park, Hyojung, Ruobing Li, Chun Yang, Josh Grimm, and Lance Porter. 2023. The Role of Media in Addressing Opioid Use Disorder: Examining Causal Attributions and Emotions as Mediators of Media Influence on Stigma and Policy Support. *Journal of Health Communication* 28 (12): 835–845. https://doi.org/10.1080/10810730.2023.2270450.

Patel, Kant, and Mark E. Rushefsky. 2022. The Opioid Epidemic in the United States: Missed Opportunities and Policy Failures. Routledge, Taylor & Francis Group.

Perry, Brea L., Bernice A. Pescosolido, and Anne C. Krendl. 2020. The Unique Nature of Public Stigma toward Non-medical Prescription Opioid Use and Dependence: A National Study. *Addiction* 115 (12): 2317–2326. https://doi.org/10.1111/add.15069.

Rummans, Teresa A., M. Caroline Burton, and Nancy L. Dawson. 2018. How Good Intentions Contributed to Bad Outcomes: The Opioid Crisis. *Mayo Clinic Proceedings* 93 (3): 344–350. https://doi.org/10.1016/j.mayocp.2017.12.020.

Spitz, Lindsey. 2020. Poppies, Pain, and Public Health Crises: How Pain Treatment Shaped the American Opioid Epidemic. *Scientific Kenyon: The Neuroscience Edition* 4 (1): 81–88.

Tsai, Alexander C., Mathew V. Kiang, Michael L. Barnett, et al. 2019. Stigma as a Fundamental Hindrance to the United States Opioid Overdose Crisis Response. *PLOS Medicine* 16 (11): e1002969. https://doi.org/10.1371/journal.pmed.1002969.

U. S. Centers for Disease Control and Prevention. 2025. *Understanding the Opioid Overdose Epidemic.* https://www.cdc.gov/overdose-prevention/about/understanding-the-opioid-overdose-epidemic.html#:~:text=The%20rise%20in%20opioid%20overdose,2.

Woodcock, Janet. 2013. Purdue pharma L. P.; Withdrawal of Approval of a New Drug Application for Oxycontin. FDA-2013-N-0883. The Food and Drug Administration. https://www.federalregister.gov/documents/2013/08/07/2013-18694/purdue-pharma-lp-withdrawal-of-approval-of-a-new-drug-application-for-oxycontin.

World Health Organization. 2001. *The World Health Report: 2002: Mental Health: New Understanding, New Hope*. World Health Organization. https://iris.who.int/handle/10665/42390.

PART I

Communicating Chronic Pain, Opioid Use Disorder, Treatment, and Harm Reduction

CHAPTER 2

The Role of Language in Stigmatizing Opioid Use Disorder

Övgü Kaynak, Christopher R. Whipple, and Nathan E. Kruis

2.1 Introduction

Despite a concerted effort to increase the use of person-first, non-stigmatizing language in the addiction field and the larger community, the use of stigmatizing language to describe the opioid crisis and people using opioids persists. Stigma is a veritable obstacle to a coordinated response to the opioid crisis (Tsai et al. 2019). Stigma toward opioids and the people who use them is a recognized barrier to opioid use disorder (OUD) treatment initiation and completion, the availability of harm reduction strategies (e.g., opioid overdose prevention centers, syringe services programs, fentanyl test strips, and naloxone distribution), and the use of effective medications for OUD (e.g., methadone and buprenorphine; Crapanzano

Ö. Kaynak (✉) • C. R. Whipple
Social Sciences and Psychology, Penn State Harrisburg, Middletown, PA, USA
e-mail: oik101@psu.edu; crw5586@psu.edu

N. E. Kruis
Criminal Justice, Penn State Altoona, Altoona, PA, USA
e-mail: nek132@psu.edu

X. Cao (ed.), *Fighting the Opioid Crisis with Communication*,
https://doi.org/10.1007/978-3-032-31162-7_2

et al. 2018; Wakeman and Rich 2018; Hanson et al. 2024). Further, people who stigmatize opioid users favor punitive measures over treatment and show lower levels of support for public health-oriented strategies to tackle the opioid crisis (Kennedy-Hendricks et al. 2017; Taylor et al. 2021; Kaynak et al. 2022). One way stigma is perpetuated is through language. Stigmatizing language used by the general public and healthcare practitioners to describe the opioid crisis and the people who use opioids is dehumanizing, resulting in bias and discrimination that further isolate those who need treatment (Werder et al. 2022). The latest data (National Center for Health Statistics 2026) show opioids were involved in 64% of the 69, 973 deaths from drug overdoses in the U.S. in 2025, highlighting the urgency to positively impact the way society communicates about and addresses the opioid crisis. Hence, this chapter will (1) describe and contextualize stigma and stigmatizing language as they relate to OUD, (2) synthesize the current literature on OUD stigma and language with a focus on how stigmatizing language exacerbates the stigma of individuals who use opioids, and (3) summarize recommendations for and examples of identifying and replacing stigmatizing language used by the general public and in treatment settings.

2.2 Understanding the Stigma of Opioid Use Disorder

In one of the first conceptualizations of stigma, Erving Goffman (1963) linked the concept to a discrediting attribute that distinguishes individuals from others and results in their social devaluation—which he famously referred to as having a "spoiled identity." Contemporary stigma theorists have expanded this definition to include labeling, status loss, and discrimination (Link and Phelan 2001). In the context of substance use, stigma refers to holding "negative attitudes and stereotypes" about substance use disorders (SUD) which can serve as barriers to treatment and lead to negative behavioral responses (National Institute on Drug Abuse 2022). SUD, including OUD, have long been recognized as stigmatized conditions (Room et al. 2001; Taylor et al. 2021). This stigmatization can occur at the interpersonal (e.g., social stigma), intrapersonal (e.g., self-stigma), and societal levels (e.g., structural stigma) with research showing that each type leads to negative health outcomes for people who use opioids (Luoma et al. 2008; Corrigan et al. 2009; Hatzenbuehler and Link 2014; Pescosolido and Martin 2015).

It is important to understand the nuances between variants of stigma and where they occur. Stigmas at the interpersonal levels include social, courtesy, and provider-based stigmas. Social stigma, also known as "public" stigma, refers to stigma held and/or enacted upon by members of the public toward stigmatized groups (Corrigan et al. 2017); some examples include community members purposefully excluding those with lived substance use experiences from community events or banding together to prevent treatment facilities from being built near their homes (Kruis et al. 2024). Courtesy stigma occurs when this stigmatization extends to those associated with "marked groups," including family members and friends (Pescosolido and Martin 2015). One example would be when a family member is socially rejected due to their loved one's OUD. Provider-based stigma refers to stigma enacted upon by professionals who have occupationally driven encounters with marginalized groups (Kruis and Merlo 2021). One example would be a physician prescribing antiretroviral drugs in lower doses to HIV-positive people who use drugs intravenously compared to HIV-positive patients who do not use drugs intravenously due to a belief that the former are more "blameworthy" in contracting the disease. Another example would be a police officer or Emergency Medical Technician (EMT) being unwilling to administer naloxone to someone who experienced an opioid overdose due to a belief that such individuals "deserve" to suffer any adverse consequences associated with their substance use. Social, courtesy and provider-based stigmas of people using opioids are rooted in perceptions of dangerousness, blameworthiness, and fatalism of opioid use, as well as a desire for greater social distance from opioid users (Kruis and Merlo 2021). Those who place greater levels of stigma onto opioid users view them as threatening public safety, deserving of adverse consequences associated with opioid use, and perceive OUD as a condition that most will never overcome. They do not want to be around opioid users and make efforts to avoid social—and professional—interactions with them.

Stigma at the intrapersonal level is referred to as self-stigma. In the context of opioid stigma, self-stigma involves the acceptance and internalization of "stereotypes and prejudice" about opioid users and OUD by those who use the drugs (Pescosolido and Martin 2015; Corrigan 2016; Kaynak et al. 2022). It is the process of one shaming, guilting, and "othering" themself due to their own history of opioid use, and suffering negative consequences (e.g., shame) as a result. Societal-level stigma (also known as "structural" or "institutional" stigma), on the other hand, refers to "prejudice and discrimination by policies, laws and constitutional practices" (Crapanzano et al. 2018; Wakeman and Rich 2018; Hanson et al. 2024). Examples include the criminalization of opioid misuse and subsequent laws that restrict access to social benefits for people convicted of felony drug possession, including access to welfare benefits, educational funding, employment opportunities, and voting rights.

Stigma toward opioids and the people who use them is a recognized barrier to OUD treatment initiation and completion, the availability of harm reduction strategies, and the use of effective medications for OUD (Crapanzano et al. 2018; Wakeman and Rich 2018; Hanson et al. 2024). For instance, social, provider-based, and self-stigmas of OUD have all been found to be associated with misconceptions of and negative attitudes toward the use of pharmacotherapy to treat OUD and lower support for policies designed to enhance treatment access (Kruis et al. 2021; Stone et al. 2021; Dickson-Gomez et al. 2022; Kaynak et al. 2022; dela Cruz et al. 2023). Specifically, provider-based stigma has been shown to influence the use of medications for opioid use disorder (MOUD; e.g., methadone, buprenorphine and naltrexone) in treatment settings and lower the levels of care first responders are willing to provide to those who experience an opioid overdose (Madden 2019; Priest et al. 2020; Kruis and Merlo 2021; Dickson-Gomez et al. 2022; Wood et al. 2022; Carl et al. 2023). At the same time, studies have documented the presence of stigma among treatment providers, and many individuals with OUD have reported experiencing stigma at the hands of clinicians (Stone et al. 2021; McLean et al. 2024). This stigma has been found to delay patients from initiating treatment, influence MOUD dosage and tapering, and ultimately negatively affect treatment outcomes (Dickson-Gomez et al. 2022; Pinhal et al. 2024).

2.3 Language and Stigma

Stigma is reinforced and expressed through the language we use. Stigmatizing language used to describe the opioid crisis and opioid users is often dehumanizing and discriminatory (McGinty et al. 2018; Ashford et al. 2019d). Such language can serve as a vehicle to transmit bias against individuals with OUD, shape perceptions and behavior related to these individuals, and impact OUD treatment and policy support (Ashford et al. 2019d; Park et al. 2021). Link and Phelan (2001) considered labeling (that is, using stigmatizing terms to describe people with OUD) the first step in the stigmatization process. Stigmatizing terms such as "addict" and "junkie" are believed to "[elicit] negative associations, punitive attitudes, and individual blame," making people who use drugs appear to be "the" problem rather than someone who "has" a problem (National Institute on Drug Abuse 2021). Indeed, researchers have found that words such as "addict" and "substance abuser" used in substance use treatment communities have negative connotations and are associated with implicit and explicit biases (Ashford et al. 2018). Stigmatizing words also induce negative emotions in people. For example, the word "abuse" has an emotional valence rating similar to that of words such as "homicide" and "rape," which suggests that the word "abuse" often evokes negative emotional reactions from people (Warriner et al. 2013). However, as Zwick et al. (2020) point out, "abuse" in the context of "child abuse" may merit such a negative reaction, but referring to a person with an SUD as having an "abuse problem" often evokes a negative emotional reaction that may not be warranted. As such, stigmatizing words used to describe the opioid crisis can influence public perceptions about the crisis and opioid users. Not only do they elicit negative emotions, but stigmatizing words imply that people are responsible for their addiction and thus deserve the negative consequences that come from substance use (Smith 2007). Stigmatizing language makes substance use the dominant social label attached to people who use drugs, further perpetuating misconceptions, stereotypes, and biases. There is much more to people who use drugs than their substance use history. These individuals can be parents, siblings, friends, neighbors, and co-workers, just like anyone else, and as such, they should not be defined merely by their substance use.

In addition to the stigmatizing terms used to describe people with OUD, there are more subtle ways language is used to perpetuate stigma. For example, evidence-based harm reduction strategies like needle exchange programs and naloxone distribution are labeled as "enabling" despite their demonstrated medical effectiveness (Wakeman 2019). Using words like "enabling" to describe harm reduction strategies shifts public focus to continued drug consumption from the strategies' demonstrated health benefits for people using drugs, such as reduced overdose risk and increased access to medical treatment (Vearrier 2019). Generally speaking, stigmatizing language may fall under one of several categories: language used to describe people with OUD, language used to describe behaviors of people with OUD, and language used to describe medications for OUD.

2.3.1 *Language Used to Describe People with OUD*

Stigmatizing terms that are used to describe people with OUD include "drug or substance user" or "abuser" (Kelly et al. 2010; Scholten et al. 2017; Ashford et al. 2018; Ashford et al., 2019c, d; National Institute on Drug Abuse 2021; Ho et al. 2022), "addict" or "former addict" (Scholten et al. 2017; Ashford et al. 2018; Goodyear et al. 2018; National Institute on Drug Abuse 2021; Ho et al. 2022), "drug seeker" (Ho et al. 2022), "user" (National Institute on Drug Abuse 2021), "junkie" (Scholten et al. 2017; Ashford et al. 2019c; National Institute on Drug Abuse 2021), and "crackhead" or "druggie" (Burgess et al. 2021). Stigmatizing language used to describe people with OUD generally conflates the disorder with a person's identity. As such, rather than referring to OUD as a disorder that the person experiences, these words or phrases identify the person solely based on their disorder. The media has consistently perpetuated substance use stigma through the use of stigmatizing language to describe people with OUD. In a review of 6399 news articles published on the opioid crisis over a 10-year period, almost half contained stigmatizing language when referring to people with OUD (McGinty et al. 2019).

2.3.2 *Language Used to Describe the Behaviors of People with OUD*

Stigmatizing language used to describe the behaviors of people with OUD often relies on outdated terminology for SUD or reflects negative evaluations of people with OUD. Outdated words such as "addiction," "abuse" (Scholten et al. 2017; National Institute on Drug Abuse 2021; Ho et al. 2022), or "relapse" (Ashford et al. 2018) may be considered stigmatizing, pejorative, and imprecise in how they describe substance-related disorders and associated behaviors (Scholten et al. 2017). For example, the term "recurrence" is typically used by the medical community to refer to the return of a disease after a period of improvement or remission, but the word "relapse" is used to denote the return of opioid misuse. The Latin root of the word "relapse" literally means "slipped back," which implies a lack of control of the individual in recovery and, therefore, is stigmatizing and pejorative. Language that suggests choice or culpability in OUD includes specific words such as "habit" (National Institute on Drug Abuse 2021), or statements implying that people with OUD are choosing to continue their disorder (e.g., "they're a lost cause. Oh, they're not going to get anywhere" [Francia et al. 2023, 4]). Other words or statements suggest that moral failure contributes to the disorder such as the words "clean/dirty" used to refer to whether a test came back positive or negative for substance use (Scholten et al. 2017) and the statements attaching moral- or character-based attributions to the disorder (e.g., "You hear the word 'addict' and you automatically think a homeless person, a jobless person, a broke person, someone that is stealing, someone that doesn't care about their kids" [Judd et al. 2023b, 473]). These words or expressions often suggest a moral model of addiction (Frank and Nagel 2017) in which people develop OUD because they are weak, selfish, and flawed. Moreover, when people with OUD seek medication (e.g., antibiotics) for illness, they are often described by healthcare professionals as "drug seeking" once their addiction history is revealed (Burgess et al. 2021).

2.3.3 Language Used to Describe Treatment for OUD

Lastly, stigmatizing language used to describe medication for OUD may implicitly or explicitly suggest that medications for OUD are in some way supplemental and not lifesaving on their own and that these medications enable the continuation of substance use. Terms like "opioid replacement therapy" or "opioid substitution therapy" may suggest that such treatments are replacing one drug with another (Scholten et al. 2017; National Institute on Drug Abuse 2021; Ho et al. 2022). Other terms, such as "medication-assisted treatment," may indicate that, to be successful, medication must be accompanied by some other treatment (Ashford et al. 2018; National Institute on Drug Abuse 2021; Ho et al. 2022). Therapy that does not include evidence-based medication is known as "drug-free," which implies that a person who uses a medication for OUD is not actually in recovery (Olsen and Sharfstein 2014).

2.4 Consequences of Stigmatizing Language on the Health and Well-Being of People with OUD

Stigmatizing language perpetuates stigma and negatively impacts the health and well-being of individuals with OUD. Specifically, there is evidence suggesting that stigmatizing language is associated with support for incarceration over treatment and a desire for social distance from people with OUD (Kelly et al. 2010). Such language also leads people with OUD to avoid medical treatment for fear of being labeled (Judd et al. 2023b). Moreover, stigmatizing language can compromise the medical treatment people with OUD receive (Dickson-Gomez et al. 2022; Hooker et al. 2023), decrease utilization of and support for harm reduction strategies (Cortina 2013; Fomiatti et al. 2022), and undermine support for public health-oriented policies (Taylor et al. 2021; McLean et al. 2024).

Historically, people with OUD have been labeled by society in such a way as to justify their alienation or being put in prison instead of a treatment facility. For example, the "substance users" were perceived as a greater social threat and as willingly engaging in misconduct. Indeed, a survey by Ledford and colleagues found that stigmatizing terms used to label people who use opioids (e.g., opioid addict) resulted in greater perceptions of dangerousness and threat posed by these people (Ledford et al. 2022). Consequently, referring to someone as a "substance user" as opposed to someone with SUD was found to result in higher levels of public support for punishment rather than treatment (Kelly et al. 2010). Those who endorsed high levels of stigma also expressed a desire for increased social distance from people with OUD. People with OUD often encounter stigmatizing labels (e.g., crackhead, tweaker) and report that those labels had a negative impact on their willingness to seek treatment for their disorder and other medical conditions (Judd et al. 2023b). In particular, when negatively labeled by those in helping professions (i.e., nurses and law enforcement), people with OUD will actively avoid them for fear of further stigmatizing experiences.

Even when people with OUD seek out medical care, stigmatizing language can negatively influence the quality of care they receive. For example, primary care clinicians who use language that differentiates, demeans, or blames people with OUD for their disorder are less likely to prescribe MOUD like buprenorphine (Hooker et al. 2023; Dickson-Gomez et al. 2022; Stone et al. 2021). Furthermore, language that depicts MOUD as drugs (e.g., "I felt like Suboxone [buprenorphine] was trading one addiction for another"; Dickson-Gomez et al. 2022, 3) can negatively impact pharmacists' willingness to dispense MOUD and the availability and use of MOUD in carceral settings, like prisons (Komalasari et al. 2021). Francia et al. (2023), in their interviews with people with SUD and healthcare professionals, found that the use of stigmatizing language (e.g., "he's just a scumbag") that othered people with SUD communicated to staff that these people were undeserving of their time and care. Moreover, labeling people with OUD as "addicts" may negatively impact healthcare professionals' belief that these people should be prescribed pain medication. For instance, in focus groups of postpartum women, participants recounted being denied pain medication during labor (e.g., "…nurse told me I did not need any pain medication because I was on Suboxone and was a drug addict"; Burgess et al. 2021, 3).

Stigmatizing language can follow people with OUD throughout the healthcare system via documentation (e.g., medical records) that propagates stigma (e.g., dirty urine and drug-seeking), which can negatively impact medical treatment (Hoover et al. 2022; Weiner et al. 2023). For example, medical documentation that describes a patient going through opioid withdrawal in an overtly negative way (e.g., nasty person and nightmare) can result in trepidation around treating people with OUD and adversely impact patient-practitioner interactions (Francia et al. 2023). Stigmatizing language in medical charts can also impact practitioner treatment recommendations. For instance, P. Goddu (2018) and colleagues found that, when compared to medical students who read neutral medical charts, medical students who read charts that used stigmatizing language (e.g., narcotic dependent) to describe a sickle cell disease patient reported more negative attitudes toward that patient and prescribed less aggressive pain management. Finally, if people with OUD become aware of the stigmatizing language used to describe them in medical charts, it may influence treatment adherence. Being labeled as an "addict" in medical charts can shame people with OUD and result in their discontinuation of pain medications to avoid that label and its associated negative social consequences (Hoover et al. 2022).

Stigmatizing language is also associated with decreased utilization of and support for harm reduction strategies (e.g., naloxone) to prevent overdose. For example, flyers depicting children playing alongside discarded syringes and denouncing "junkies and drug pushers" have been used by opponents of safe injection facilities in Canada (Cortina 2013). This stigmatizing language is used to reinforce a "war on drugs" position and dehumanize people with OUD who need help. In a qualitative study of health professionals and people who use opioids in Australia, Fomiatti et al. (2022) reported that fear of discrimination from health professionals influenced the willingness of opioid users to get naloxone from their doctors. A person who used opioids reported not asking their doctor about naloxone because they were afraid that "people might think (they're) a druggie" if they carried around naloxone (Fomiatti et al. 2022, 149). A pharmacist indicated that many pharmacies choose not to stock naloxone "because they don't want to … invite the wrong crowd into the pharmacy" (Fomiatti et al. 2022, 150). In another qualitative study (Wild et al. 2021), beliefs about the disease model of addiction affected support for harm reduction strategies in Canada. People who scored higher on beliefs that addiction is a chronic disorder for which the only true treatment is abstinence (e.g., "There are only two possibilities for an alcoholic or drug addict-permanent abstinence or death" [Wild et al. 2021, 7]) reported lower support for harm reduction strategies.

Stigmatizing language is also associated with less support for other public health-related policies, beyond access to harm reduction strategies. Language that disregards OUD as a medical condition (e.g., "Opioid use disorder/addiction is a moral failing") or OUD medication as legitimate treatments (e.g., "Medication for OUD is a hoax") is associated with less support for public health-oriented policies, such as expanding Medicaid insurance benefits, increasing government spending for SUD intervention, and providing access to MOUD in jail or prison (Taylor et al. 2021). In qualitative interviews with OUD treatment providers and people who supervise individuals with OUD in the criminal justice system, the association between stigmatizing language and reduced support for treatment was further supported (McLean et al. 2024). Specifically, language used by criminal justice professionals that writes individuals off as "just a junkie" and characterizes addiction as a moral failure was cited as a reason why justice-involved individuals with OUD avoided treatment or concealed their OUD from treatment providers ("I think there's a stigma among people who don't…really understand what those folks are going through on a mental health level. That think that they are just a junkie, or you know, they made that choice for themselves" [McLean et al. 2024, 8]). Labels like "junkie" perpetuate the idea that OUD is a choice and make it easier for criminal justice professionals to marginalize people with OUD as criminals deserving of punishment rather than treatment. This results in arcane institutional regulation policies that delay initiation of MOUD and deter justice-involved people with OUD from enrolling in treatment while incarcerated (McLean et al. 2024).

While attitudes and beliefs about stigmatizing language among people with OUD are not well-studied, there is evidence suggesting that some individuals with lived experience reappropriate stigmatizing language through self-labeling (Galinsky et al. 2013). This practice may serve as a protective response to stigma, promoting psychological empowerment and social cohesion, potentially buffering against some of the harmful effects that stigmatizing language can have on health and well-being. While people in OUD recovery may not consider terms like "addict" to be stigmatizing when they use the word themselves (Ashford et al. 2019a, b), there is enough evidence to show that when someone is referred to as an "addict," they are generally viewed more negatively. Thus, while people with OUD may call themselves "addicts," they prefer that others with no lived experience use non-stigmatizing language (Pivovarova and Stein 2019). Even when people in recovery do not consider certain terms to be stigmatizing, their internalization of these negative labels is evident in the way they describe people without SUD as being "normal" and their desire to keep their substance use history secret (Blyth et al. 2023). When stigmatizing language is used by the general public, people with OUD can experience shame and negative self-perception, leading to avoidance of treatments for OUD to avoid the label (Woods and Joseph 2015). Internalizing stigmatizing language used by the public can also result in fatalism about the ability to recover ("All we've ever heard is, 'Oh, you're an addict. Oh, you're a drunk.' 'Oh, you're an alcoholic, that's all you'll ever be'"; Judd et al. 2023a, 473). Internalizing fatalistic messaging (e.g., "hopeless to recover" and "doomed to fail") in turn can lead to substance use treatment avoidance and even a return to excessive substance use (Slomski 2021).

2.5 Recommendations to Address Bias and Stigma in Language

Considering the harm that stigmatizing language can have on people with OUD, several recommendations have been made to change the way we communicate about the opioid crisis and people who use opioids, including using person-first language, identifying and replacing stigmatizing terms, and including people with lived experience in OUD trainings and interventions. As discussed previously, much of the stigmatizing language used to describe people with OUD comes from implicitly labeling a person as the disorder with which they suffer. For example, referring to a person as an "addict" or a "substance abuser" highlights the person's substance use as a key aspect of their identity. On the contrary, the use of person-first language centers the person and identifies the disorder as only one aspect of the person's life (Broyles et al. 2014; Kelly et al. 2016; Ashford et al. 2019c; Volkow et al. 2021). Person-first language (e.g., individual with OUD) highlights the person's humanity first and is less likely to communicate bias. Studies have found that using person-first language in surveys can result in more benevolent and less authoritarian views of people with SUD (Baker et al. 2022). There is also support for the use of person-first language in healthcare settings. Carpenter et al. (2023) reviewed the medical records of patients with OUD who were admitted to the hospital for infections associated with injection opioid use. When patient discharge summaries used person-first language (e.g., having an SUD), patients were significantly more likely to have a documented plan for OUD treatment, compared to patients whose discharge orders included premodified nouns (e.g., addict).

In addition to using person-first language, there is a need to identify and replace stigmatizing language with non-stigmatizing language. Multiple attempts have been made by researchers to identify stigmatizing terms or phrases and to offer non-stigmatizing alternatives (Scholten et al. 2017; Ashford et al. 2019c; National Institute on Drug Abuse 2021). For example, National Institute on Drug Abuse (2021) provided a concise list of terms to avoid and alternative terms to use when talking about SUD. In addition to suggesting the use of person-first language for stigmatizing terms, they also provided a list of other stigmatizing words, with alternative words and why the stigmatizing word is problematic (e.g., replacing dirty with testing positive). Discouraging the use of stigmatizing terms and phrases and educating people on non-stigmatizing alternatives may result in lower levels of perceived stigma toward people with OUD. For example, a recent randomized control trial tested OUD stigma-focused visual messaging and short narrative vignettes denouncing stigmatizing language, championing person-first language, and emphasizing effective treatment tailored to healthcare providers (Kennedy-Hendricks et al. 2022). Participants in the *Words Matter* frame condition were exposed to visual and narrative messaging discouraging stigmatizing language and encouraging the use of non-stigmatizing language when working with patients with OUD. When compared to nonexposed participants, participants exposed to the *Words Matter* frame were significantly more willing to have a person with OUD marry into the family (i.e., a measure of social distance) and had a significantly higher level of warmth toward people with OUD (Kennedy-Hendricks et al. 2022). These findings suggest that among healthcare providers, employing messages about non-stigmatizing language reduced stigma toward people with OUD.

Lastly, including people with lived experiences in interventions may impact the use of stigmatizing language and help increase empathy and understanding toward individuals with OUD (Slomski 2021). Many of the stigmatizing words and phrases used to describe people with OUD connote negative and biased evaluations of people with OUD (e.g., these people are just addicts, dangerous or criminals, or will never get better). Generally, contact-based strategies aim to change entrenched biases through direct contact with people from the stigmatized group (Livingston et al. 2012). In its simplest form, including a person with lived experience can impact the language one uses to describe someone with an SUD through the risk of social disapproval (e.g., a resident presenting a case study during grand rounds and referring to a patient as "an alcoholic admitted again" vs. correcting themselves to say a patient with "alcohol use disorder"; [Slomski 2021, 1468]). However, the type of contact (i.e., negative vs. positive) may be important when the aim is to reduce stigmatizing views. For example, a study found that using an imagined contact exercise to prime participants with positive empathy resulted in lower levels of reported stigma toward people with OUD (Clinton and Pollini 2021). To this end, contact-based strategies can use recovery success stories to decrease stigmatizing attitudes by humanizing people with OUD and promoting perspective-taking among people with no experience with addiction (Judd et al. 2023a). Such stories may combat the negative, attributional, and fatalistic attitudes about people with OUD. An example of a promising intervention that incorporates a contact-based strategy is *Life Unites Us,* a social media campaign that centers on testimonial videos from individuals in recovery from OUD and SUD (Bonnevie et al. 2022; Kaynak et al. 2022; Whipple et al. 2024). The campaign was designed to target stigma in the public to correct stereotypes, bring the public into contact with individuals with OUD through testimonials, and invite the public to actively support individuals with OUD. In addition to the testimonials, the campaign also utilizes static messages to increase public knowledge about language that stigmatizes vs. empowers (e.g., "Language matters. Use empowering language like, 'person with an OUD' instead of hurtful words like 'addict' or 'junkie'" or say "people with OUD get better"). All components of the campaign, from campaign messaging to community training and resources, include information on appropriate non-stigmatizing language to use when referring to people with OUD. After a year of the campaign, an evaluation revealed that when compared to those who did not view the campaign, those who viewed the campaign reported more positive attitudes toward people with OUD (Whipple et al. 2024).

2.6 Conclusions

Existing research on the relation between language and OUD stigma suggests that negative emotions and beliefs are associated with stigmatizing language. The use of stigmatizing language may influence overall evaluations of people with OUD, as well as specific evaluations of their responsibility for their disorder and their perceived dangerousness. When people with OUD are labeled using stigmatizing terminology (e.g., substance abusers and opioid addicts), they are more likely to be viewed as bad, responsible for their OUD, dangerous, and subsequently avoided. Beyond negative evaluations of people with OUD by others, stigmatizing language is associated with negative self-evaluations of people with OUD. Often, the language used to describe OUD and people with OUD leads to internalized or self-stigma among people with OUD. Such internalization can manifest in increased desire to conceal one's OUD, fear of discrimination from others, and fatalistic attitudes about their own continued use and ability to recover. To address bias and stigma in language, it is important to use person-first language, identify and replace stigmatizing terms, and encourage empathy and understanding through lived experiences. It is also crucial to implement and support interventions that promote person-first, non-stigmatizing language and raise awareness about the challenges and successes of treatment and long-term recovery. By doing so, we can foster a more empathetic and understanding society, ultimately reducing stigma and improving health outcomes for people with OUD.

References

Ashford, Robert D., Austin M. Brown, and Brenda Curtis. 2018. Substance Use, Recovery, and Linguistics: The Impact of Word Choice on Explicit and Implicit Bias. *Drug and Alcohol Dependence* 189:131–138. https://doi.org/10.1016/j.drugalcdep.2018.05.005.

Ashford, Robert D., Austin M. Brown, Arielle Ashford, and Brenda Curtis. 2019a. Recovery Dialects: A Pilot Study of Stigmatizing and Nonstigmatizing Label Use by Individuals in Recovery from Substance Use Disorders. *Experimental and Clinical Psychopharmacology* 27 (6): 530–535. https://doi.org/10.1037/pha0000286.

Ashford, Robert D., Austin M. Brown, Jessica McDaniel, and Brenda Curtis. 2019b. Biased Labels: An Experimental Study of Language and Stigma among Individuals in Recovery and Health Professionals. *Substance Use & Misuse* 54 (8): 1376–1384. https://doi.org/10.1080/10826084.2019.1581221.

Ashford, Robert D., Austin M. Brown, and Brenda Curtis. 2019c. Expanding Language Choices to Reduce Stigma: A Delphi Study of Positive and Negative Terms in Substance Use and Recovery. *Health Education* 119 (1): 51–62. https://doi.org/10.1108/HE-03-2018-0017.

Ashford, Robert D., Austin M. Brown, and Brenda Curtis. 2019d. 'Abusing Addiction': Our Language Still isn't Good Enough. *Alcoholism Treatment Quarterly* 37 (2): 257–272. https://doi.org/10.1080/07347324.2018.1513777.

Baker, Emily A., Mark Hamilton, Danielle Culpepper, Grace McCune, and Gabriella Silone. 2022. The Effect of Person-first Language on Attitudes toward People with Addiction. *Journal of Addictions & Offender Counseling* 43 (1): 38–49. https://doi.org/10.1002/jaoc.12102.

Blyth, Sophia H., Kiefer Cowie, Jordan Jurinsky, and Emily A. Hennessy. 2023. A Qualitative Examination of Social Identity and Stigma among Adolescents Recovering from Alcohol or Drug Use. *Addictive Behaviors Reports* 18:100505. https://doi.org/10.1016/j.abrep.2023.100505.

Bonnevie, Erika, Övgü Kaynak, Christopher R. Whipple, et al. 2022. Life Unites Us: A Novel Approach to Addressing Opioid Use Disorder Stigma. *Health Education Journal* 81 (3): 312–324. https://doi.org/10.1177/00178969221077409.

Broyles, Lauren M., Ingrid A. Binswanger, Jennifer A. Jenkins, et al. 2014. Confronting Inadvertent Stigma and Pejorative Language in Addiction Scholarship: A Recognition and Response. *Substance Abuse* 35 (3): 217–221. https://doi.org/10.1080/08897077.2014.930372.

Burgess, Amanda, Emily Bauer, Shane Gallagher, et al. 2021. Experiences of Stigma among Individuals in Recovery from Opioid Use Disorder in a Rural Setting: A Qualitative Analysis. *Journal of Substance Abuse Treatment* 130:108488. https://doi.org/10.1016/j.jsat.2021.108488.

Carl, Alexis, Emily Pasman, Michael J. Broman, Jamey J. Lister, Elizabeth Agius, and Stella M. Resko. 2023. Experiences of Healthcare and Substance Use Treatment Provider-Based Stigma among Patients Receiving Methadone. *Drug and Alcohol Dependence Reports* 6:100138. https://doi.org/10.1016/j.dadr.2023.100138.

Carpenter, Joseph E., Jillian Catalanotti, Melissa Notis, et al. 2023. Use of Nonstigmatizing Language Is Associated with Improved Outcomes in Hospitalized People Who Inject Drugs. *Journal of Hospital Medicine* 18 (8): 670–676. https://doi.org/10.1002/jhm.13146.

Clinton, Alex J., and Robin A. Pollini. 2021. Using Positive Empathy Interventions to Reduce Stigma toward People Who Inject Drugs. *Frontiers in Psychology* 12:616729. https://doi.org/10.3389/fpsyg.2021.616729.

Corrigan, Patrick W. 2016. Lessons Learned from Unintended Consequences about Erasing the Stigma of Mental Illness. *World Psychiatry* 15 (1): 67–73. https://doi.org/10.1002/wps.20295.

Corrigan, Patrick W., Sachiko A. Kuwabara, and John O'Shaughnessy. 2009. The Public Stigma of Mental Illness and Drug Addiction: Findings from a Stratified Random Sample. *Journal of Social Work* 9 (2): 139–147. https://doi.org/10.1177/1468017308101818.

Corrigan, Patrick W., Georg Schomerus, Valery Shuman, et al. 2017. Developing a Research Agenda for Understanding the Stigma of Addictions Part I: Lessons from the Mental Health Stigma Literature. *The American Journal on Addictions* 26 (1): 59–66. https://doi.org/10.1111/ajad.12458.

Cortina, Sandra C. 2013. Stigmatizing Harm Reduction Through Language: A Case Study Into the Use of 'Addict' and Opposition to Supervised Injection Sites in Canada. *Journal of Addictions Nursing* 24 (2): 102–107. https://doi.org/10.1097/jan.0b013e3182929466.

Crapanzano, Kathleen, Rebecca Hammarlund, Bilal Ahmad, Natalie Hunsinger, and Rumneet Kullar. 2018. The Association between Perceived Stigma and Substance Use Disorder Treatment Outcomes: A Review. *Substance Abuse and Rehabilitation* 10:1–12. https://doi.org/10.2147/SAR.S183252.

Cruz, Adriane M. dela, Tara Karns-Wright, Farra Kahalnik, et al. 2023. Stigma towards Opioid Use Disorder in Primary Care Remain a Barrier to Integrating Software-Based Measurement Based Care. *BMC Psychiatry* 23 (1): 776. https://doi.org/10.1186/s12888-023-05267-w.

Dickson-Gomez, Julia, Antoinette Spector, Margaret Weeks, Carol Galletly, Madelyn McDonald, and Helena Danielle Green Montaque. 2022. 'You're not Supposed to be on it Forever': Medications to Treat Opioid Use Disorder (MOUD) Related Stigma among Drug Treatment Providers and People who Use Opioids. *Substance Abuse: Research and Treatment* 16:11782218221103859. https://doi.org/10.1177/11782218221103859.

Fomiatti, Renae, Adrian Farrugia, Suzanne Fraser, Robyn Dwyer, Joanne Neale, and John Strang. 2022. Addiction Stigma and the Production of Impediments to Take-Home Naloxone Uptake. *Health: An Interdisciplinary Journal for the Social Study of Health, Illness and Medicine* 26 (2): 139–161. https://doi.org/10.1177/1363459320925863.

Francia, Leanne, Tina Lam, Amelia Berg, et al. 2023. Alcohol and other Drug Use: A Qualitative Exploration of Staff and Patient's Experiences of Language Use as a Means of Stigma Communication in Hospital and Primary Care Settings. *Journal of Substance Use and Addiction Treatment* 149:209050. https://doi.org/10.1016/j.josat.2023.209050.

Frank, Lily E., and Saskia K. Nagel. 2017. Addiction and Moralization: The Role of the Underlying Model of Addiction. *Neuroethics* 10 (1): 129–139. https://doi.org/10.1007/s12152-017-9307-x.

Galinsky, Adam D., Cynthia S. Wang, Jennifer A. Whitson, Eric M. Anicich, Kurt Hugenberg, and Galen V. Bodenhausen. 2013. The Reappropriation of Stigmatizing Labels: The Reciprocal Relationship between Power and Self-

Labeling. *Psychological Science* 24 (10): 2020–2029. https://doi.org/10.1177/0956797613482943.

Goddu, Anna P., Katie J. O'Conor, Sophie Lanzkron, et al. 2018. Do Words Matter? Stigmatizing Language and the Transmission of Bias in the Medical Record. *Journal of General Internal Medicine* 33 (5): 685–691. https://doi.org/10.1007/s11606-017-4289-2.

Goffman, Erving. 1963. 1922–1982. *Stigma; Notes on the Management of Spoiled Identity*. Englewood Cliffs, N.J: Prentice-Hall, [1963]. https://search.library.wisc.edu/catalog/999472649302121.

Goodyear, Kimberly, Carolina L. Haass-Koffler, and David Chavanne. 2018. Opioid Use and Stigma: The Role of Gender, Language and Precipitating Events. *Drug and Alcohol Dependence* 185:339–346. https://doi.org/10.1016/j.drugalcdep.2017.12.037.

Hanson, Bridget L., Kari Finley, Jay Otto, Nicholas J. Ward, and Swagata Banik. 2024. Community Support for Harm Reduction and Treatment of Opioid Use Disorder. *Journal of Community Health* 49 (4): 724–731. https://doi.org/10.1007/s10900-023-01278-6.

Hatzenbuehler, Mark L., and Bruce G. Link. 2014. Introduction to the Special Issue on Structural Stigma and Health. *Social Science & Medicine* 103:1–6. https://doi.org/10.1016/j.socscimed.2013.12.017.

Ho, J. Janet, Katie F. Jones, Zachary Sager, Sarah Wakeman, and Jessica S. Merlin. 2022. De-Stigmatizing the Language of Addiction #429. *Journal of Palliative Medicine* 25 (1): 155–157. https://doi.org/10.1089/jpm.2021.0478.

Hooker, Stephanie A., A. Lauren Crain, Amy B. LaFrance, et al. 2023. A Randomized Controlled Trial of an Intervention to Reduce Stigma toward People with Opioid Use Disorder among Primary Care Clinicians. *Addiction Science & Clinical Practice* 18 (1): 10. https://doi.org/10.1186/s13722-023-00366-1.

Hoover, Kaitlyn, Steve Lockhart, Catherine Callister, Jodi Summers Holtrop, and Susan L. Calcaterra. 2022. Experiences of Stigma in Hospitals with Addiction Consultation Services: A Qualitative Analysis of Patients' and Hospital-Based Providers' Perspectives. *Journal of Substance Abuse Treatment* 138:108708. https://doi.org/10.1016/j.jsat.2021.108708.

Judd, Hailey, Cristian L. Meier, Ashley C. Yaugher, Emma Campbell, and Kandice Atisme-Bevins. 2023a. Opioid Use Disorder Stigma Reduction through Story Telling Narrative and Sharing: A Qualitative Review and Lessons Learned. *International Journal of Mental Health and Addiction* 21:468–483. https://doi.org/10.1007/s11469-021-00606-y.

Judd, Hailey, Ashley C. Yaugher, Sydney O'Shay, and Cristian L. Meier. 2023b. Understanding Stigma through the Lived Experiences of People with Opioid Use Disorder. *Drug and Alcohol Dependence* 249:110873. https://doi.org/10.1016/j.drugalcdep.2023.110873.

Kaynak, Övgü, Christopher R. Whipple, Erika Bonnevie, et al. 2022. The Opioid Epidemic and the State of Stigma: A Pennsylvania Statewide Survey. *Substance Use & Misuse* 57 (7): 1120–1130. https://doi.org/10.1080/10826084.2022.2064506.

Kelly, John F., Sarah J. Dow, and Cara Westerhoff. 2010. Does Our Choice of Substance-Related Terms Influence Perceptions of Treatment Need? An Empirical Investigation with Two Commonly Used Terms. *Journal of Drug Issues* 40 (4): 805–818. https://doi.org/10.1177/002204261004000403.

Kelly, John F., Richard Saitz, and Sarah Wakeman. 2016. Language, Substance Use Disorders, and Policy: The Need to Reach Consensus on an 'Addictionary'. *Alcoholism Treatment Quarterly* 34 (1): 116–123.

Kennedy-Hendricks, Alene, Colleen L. Barry, Sarah E. Gollust, Margaret E. Ensminger, Margaret S. Chisolm, and Emma E. McGinty. 2017. Social Stigma toward Persons with Prescription Opioid Use Disorder: Associations with Public Support for Punitive and Public Health–Oriented Policies. *Psychiatric Services* 68 (5): 462–469. https://doi.org/10.1176/appi.ps.201600056.

Kennedy-Hendricks, Alene, Emma E. McGinty, Amber Summers, Susan Krenn, Michael I. Fingerhood, and Colleen L. Barry. 2022. Effect of Exposure to Visual Campaigns and Narrative Vignettes on Addiction Stigma among Health Care Professionals: A Randomized Clinical Trial. *JAMA Network Open* 5 (2): e2146971. https://doi.org/10.1001/jamanetworkopen.2021.46971.

Komalasari, Rita, Sarah Wilson, and Sally Haw. 2021. A Systematic Review of Qualitative Evidence on Barriers to and Facilitators of the Implementation of Opioid Agonist Treatment (OAT) Programmes in Prisons. *International Journal of Drug Policy* 87:102978. https://doi.org/10.1016/j.drugpo.2020.102978.

Kruis, Nathan E., and Alida V. Merlo. 2021. A Preliminary Assessment of Stigma in Law Enforcement Officers' Responses to Opioid Overdoses. *Journal of Drug Issues* 51 (2): 301–322. https://doi.org/10.1177/0022042620974076.

Kruis, Nathan E., Katherine McLean, and Payton Perry. 2021. Exploring First Responders' Perceptions of Medication for Addiction Treatment: Does Stigma Influence Attitudes? *Journal of Substance Abuse Treatment* 131:108485. https://doi.org/10.1016/j.jsat.2021.108485.

Kruis, Nathan E., Övgü Kaynak, Christopher Whipple, Erica Saylor, and Weston Kensinger. 2024. Addiction Frameworks, Social Stigma, and NIMBY Syndrome: Examining Barriers to Responding to the Opioid Crisis. *Contemporary Drug Problems* 51 (1): 3–24. https://doi.org/10.1177/00914509241231821.

Ledford, Victoria, Jungkyu Rhys Lim, Kang Namkoong, Junhan Chen, and Yan Qin. 2022. The Influence of Stigmatizing Messages on Danger Appraisal: Examining the Model of Stigma Communication for Opioid-Related Stigma, Policy Support, and Related Outcomes. *Health Communication* 37 (14): 1765–1777. https://doi.org/10.1080/10410236.2021.1920710.

Link, Bruce G., and Jo C. Phelan. 2001. Conceptualizing Stigma. *Annual Review of Sociology* 27:363–385.

Livingston, James D., Teresa Milne, Mei Lan Fang, and Erica Amari. 2012. The Effectiveness of Interventions for Reducing Stigma Related to Substance Use Disorders: A Systematic Review. *Addiction* 107 (1): 39–50. https://doi.org/10.1111/j.1360-0443.2011.03601.x.

Luoma, Jason B., Barbara S. Kohlenberg, Steven C. Hayes, Kara Bunting, and Alyssa K. Rye. 2008. Reducing Self-Stigma in Substance Abuse through Acceptance and Commitment Therapy: Model, Manual Development, and Pilot Outcomes. *Addiction Research & Theory* 16 (2): 149–165. https://doi.org/10.1080/16066350701850295.

Madden, Erin Fanning. 2019. Intervention Stigma: How Medication-Assisted Treatment Marginalizes Patients and Providers. *Social Science & Medicine* 232:324–331. https://doi.org/10.1016/j.socscimed.2019.05.027.

McGinty, Emma E., Bernice Pescosolido, Alene Kennedy-Hendricks, and Colleen L. Barry. 2018. Communication Strategies to Counter Stigma and Improve Mental Illness and Substance Use Disorder Policy. *Psychiatric Services* 69 (2): 136–146. https://doi.org/10.1176/appi.ps.201700076.

McGinty, Emma E., Elizabeth M. Stone, Alene Kennedy-Hendricks, and Colleen L. Barry. 2019. Stigmatizing Language in News Media Coverage of the Opioid Epidemic: Implications for Public Health. *Preventive Medicine* 124:110–114. https://doi.org/10.1016/j.ypmed.2019.03.018.

McLean, Katherine, Jennifer Murphy, and Nathan Kruis. 2024. 'I Think We're Getting Better but We're Still Not There': Provider-Based Stigma and Perceived Barriers to Care for People Who Use Opioids (PWUO). *Journal of Substance Use and Addiction Treatment* 159:209270. https://doi.org/10.1016/j.josat.2023.209270.

National Center for Health Statistics, Center for Disease Control. 2026. U.S. Overdose Deaths Decrease for Third Consecutive Year in 2025. May 16. https://www.cdc.gov/nchs/pressroom/releases/20260513.html

National Institute on Drug Abuse. 2021. Words Matter—Terms to Use and Avoid When Talking about Addiction. https://nida.nih.gov/nidamed-medical-health-professionals/health-professions-education/words-matter-terms-to-use-avoid-when-talking-about-addiction.

National Institute on Drug Abuse. 2022. Stigma and Discrimination. https://nida.nih.gov/research-topics/stigma-discrimination.

Olsen, Yngvild, and Joshua M. Sharfstein. 2014. Confronting the Stigma of Opioid Use Disorder—and Its Treatment. *JAMA* 311 (14): 1393–1394. https://doi.org/10.1001/jama.2014.2147.

Park, Jenny, Somnath Saha, Brant Chee, Janiece Taylor, and Mary Catherine Beach. 2021. Physician Use of Stigmatizing Language in Patient Medical Records. *JAMA Network Open* 4 (7): e2117052. https://doi.org/10.1001/jamanetworkopen.2021.17052.

Pescosolido, Bernice A., and Jack K. Martin. 2015. The Stigma Complex. *Annual Review of Sociology* 41 (1): 87–116. https://doi.org/10.1146/annurev-soc-071312-145702.

Pinhal, Mélanie, Benoit Schreck, Juliette Leboucher, et al. 2024. Are the Self-Stigma and Perceived Stigma of Patients Treated with Methadone or Buprenorphine Still a Problem Fifty Years after the Marketing Authorization for Opioid Agonist Treatment? The Observational STIGMA Study. *Addiction Science & Clinical Practice* 19 (1): 74. https://doi.org/10.1186/s13722-024-00506-1.

Pivovarova, Ekaterina, and Michael D. Stein. 2019. In Their Own Words: Language Preferences of Individuals Who Use Heroin. *Addiction* 114 (10): 1785–1790. https://doi.org/10.1111/add.14699.

Priest, Kelsey C., Honora Englander, and Dennis McCarty. 2020. 'Now Hospital Leaders are Paying Attention': A Qualitative Study of Internal and External Factors Influencing Addiction Consult Services. *Journal of Substance Abuse Treatment* 110:59–65. https://doi.org/10.1016/j.jsat.2019.12.003.

Room, Robin, Jürgen Rehm, Robert T. Trotter II, Angela Paglia, and T. Bedirhan Üstün. 2001. Cross-Cultural Views on Stigma, Valuation, Parity, and Societal Values towards Disability. In *Disability and Culture: Universalism and Diversity*, edited by T. Bedirhan Üstün, Somnath Chatterji, Jerome E. Bickenbach, Robert T. Trotter II, Robin Room, and Shekhar Saxena. Hogrefe & Huber Publishers.

Scholten, Willem, Oliver Simon, Icro Maremmani, et al. 2017. Access to Treatment with Controlled Medicines Rationale and Recommendations for Neutral, Precise, and Respectful Language. *Public Health* 153:147–153. https://doi.org/10.1016/j.puhe.2017.08.021.

Slomski, Anita. 2021. The Lingua Franca of Addiction—Stigmatizing Words That Wound. *JAMA* 326 (15): 1468. https://doi.org/10.1001/jama.2021.16186.

Smith, Rachel A. 2007. Language of the Lost: An Explication of Stigma Communication. *Communication Theory* 17 (4): 462–485. https://doi.org/10.1111/j.1468-2885.2007.00307.x.

Stone, Elizabeth M., Alene Kennedy-Hendricks, Colleen L. Barry, Marcus A. Bachhuber, and Emma E. McGinty. 2021. The Role of Stigma in U.S. Primary Care Physicians' Treatment of Opioid Use Disorder. *Drug and Alcohol Dependence* 221:108627. https://doi.org/10.1016/j.drugalcdep.2021.108627.

Taylor, Bruce G., Phoebe A. Lamuda, Elizabeth Flanagan, Elizabeth Watts, Harold Pollack, and John Schneider. 2021. Social Stigma toward Persons with Opioid Use Disorder: Results from a Nationally Representative Survey of U.S. Adults. *Substance Use & Misuse* 56 (12): 1752–1764. https://doi.org/10.1080/10826084.2021.1949611.

Tsai, Alexander C., Mathew V. Kiang, Michael L. Barnett, et al. 2019. Stigma as a Fundamental Hindrance to the United States Opioid Overdose Crisis Response. *PLOS Medicine* 16 (11): e1002969. https://doi.org/10.1371/journal.pmed.1002969.

Vearrier, Laura. 2019. The Value of Harm Reduction for Injection Drug Use: A Clinical and Public Health Ethics Analysis. *Disease-a-Month* 65 (5): 119–141. https://doi.org/10.1016/j.disamonth.2018.12.002.

Volkow, Nora D., Joshua A. Gordon, and George F. Koob. 2021. Choosing Appropriate Language to Reduce the Stigma around Mental Illness and Substance Use Disorders. *Neuropsychopharmacology* 46 (13): 2230–2232. https://doi.org/10.1038/s41386-021-01069-4.

Wakeman, Sarah E. 2019. The Language of Stigma and Addiction. In *The Stigma of Addiction: An Essential Guide*, edited by Jonathan D. Avery and Joseph J. Avery. Springer International Publishing. https://doi.org/10.1007/978-3-030-02580-9.

Wakeman, Sarah E., and Josiah D. Rich. 2018. Barriers to Medications for Addiction Treatment: How Stigma Kills. *Substance Use & Misuse* 53 (2): 330–333. https://doi.org/10.1080/10826084.2017.1363238.

Warriner, Amy Beth, Victor Kuperman, and Marc Brysbaert. 2013. Norms of Valence, Arousal, and Dominance for 13,915 English Lemmas. *Behavior Research Methods* 45 (4): 1191–1207. https://doi.org/10.3758/s13428-012-0314-x.

Weiner, Scott G., Ying-Chih Lo, Aleta D. Carroll, et al. 2023. The Incidence and Disparities in Use of Stigmatizing Language in Clinical Notes for Patients with Substance Use Disorder. *Journal of Addiction Medicine* 17 (4): 424–430. https://doi.org/10.1097/adm.0000000000001145.

Werder, Karen, Alexa Curtis, Stephanie Reynolds, and Jason Satterfield. 2022. Addressing Bias and Stigma in the Language We Use with Persons with Opioid Use Disorder: A Narrative Review. *Journal of the American Psychiatric Nurses Association* 28 (1): 9–22. https://doi.org/10.1177/10783903211050121.

Whipple, Christopher R., Övgü Kaynak, Nathan E. Kruis, et al. 2024. Challenging Public Stigma: The Impact of a Statewide Social Media Campaign to Reduce Opioid Use Disorder Stigma. *Drugs: Education, Prevention and Policy* 32 (6): 596–605. https://doi.org/10.1080/09687637.2024.2416583.

Wild, T. Cameron, Jakob Koziel, Jalene Anderson-Baron, et al. 2021. Public Support for Harm Reduction: A Population Survey of Canadian Adults. *PLOS ONE* 16 (5): e0251860. https://doi.org/10.1371/journal.pone.0251860.

Wood, Claire A., Alex Duello, Jennifer Miles, et al. 2022. Acceptance of Medications for Opioid Use Disorder in Recovery Housing Programs in Missouri. *Journal of Substance Abuse Treatment* 138:108747. https://doi.org/10.1016/j.jsat.2022.108747.

Woods, Joycelyn Sue, and Herman Joseph. 2015. Stigma from the Viewpoint of the Patient. *Journal of Addictive Diseases* 34 (2–3): 238–247. https://doi.org/10.1080/10550887.2015.1059714.

Zwick, Janet, Hannah Appleseth, and Stephan Arndt. 2020. Stigma: How It Affects the Substance Use Disorder Patient. *Substance Abuse Treatment, Prevention, and Policy* 15 (1): 50. https://doi.org/10.1186/s13011-020-00288-0.

CHAPTER 3

News, Entertainment, and Social Media Portrayals of the U.S. Opioid Crisis:Stigmatizing Versus Non-stigmatizing Representations

Victoria A. Ledford

3.1 Introduction

"He found the woman slumped over the steering wheel, an empty syringe on the floorboard and her skin dulling to a purplish blue" (CBS News 2016). This sentence opened an August 2016 news article reporting a mass opioid overdose incident in Huntington, West Virginia. A tragedy for the small Appalachian city nestled in a state with the country's highest opioid overdose death rate, the incident involved 28 overdoses within 4 hours and drew national news attention. The CBS article opened with the experiences of the local emergency medical services (EMS) supervisor as he witnessed overdose after overdose in real time, providing Naloxone, a life-saving overdose response drug, to the people he found in need. It

V. A. Ledford (✉)
School of Communication and Journalism, Auburn University, Auburn, AL, USA
e-mail: vledford@auburn.edu

X. Cao (ed.), *Fighting the Opioid Crisis with Communication*,
https://doi.org/10.1007/978-3-032-31162-7_3

went on to share the stories of those who overdosed on a day that represented a turning point for the town and its response to the opioid crisis. Unfortunately, the article also included stigmatizing portrayals of people with Opioid Use Disorders (OUDs), portrayals that dehumanized people with OUDs by depicting them as something less than human, something *other*. Stigmatizing language and imagery such as "addict," "unscarred vein," and "surrounded by syringes" (CBS News 2016) are only a few examples of communication that can create harmful thoughts and actions toward people with OUDs (Ledford et al. 2022). Although news articles like this one may have aimed to draw attention to the opioid crisis and spur efforts to curb it, this type of reporting may have done more harm than good by circulating stigmatizing and dehumanizing portrayals of people with OUDs.

As opioid overdose deaths have increased in the United States (U.S.) within the last two decades (National Institute on Drug Abuse, 2024), so too has media coverage of the crisis (Hswen et al. 2020). The U.S. has one of the highest drug overdose mortality rates in the world (Y. Chen et al. 2019) and still lost more than 55,000 lives to opioid overdoses between November 2023 and November 2024, even though provisional data from 2024 suggest a decline in opioid overdose deaths compared to the previous year (CDC 2025). The opioid crisis has evolved from the rise in prescription opioid (e.g., Oxycodone, Hydrocodone, Morphine) use disorders in the early 1990s to OUDs involving synthetic opioids, like fentanyl, which now account for most opioid overdose deaths in the country, followed by heroin (CDC 2021). This rise in opioid overdose deaths in the U.S. has naturally prompted increased media attention (Hswen et al. 2020). From news media reporting (Hswen et al. 2020) to entertainment media portrayals (Oldfield et al. 2021; Gierzynski et al. 2024) to social media discourse (Jain et al. 2020), opioids occupy a significant space in the U.S. media landscape. Understanding how these three media sources portray opioids is crucial for considering the role that media play in the opioid crisis as well as for charting a path forward.

The next section of this chapter explains how media portrayals about opioids may be stigmatizing or non-stigmatizing. The chapter then reviews current research and insights on how three key media sources—news media, entertainment media, and social media—portray the U.S. opioid crisis. In doing so, the chapter considers portrayals about and by people with OUDs as well as the effects of these mediated representations on people's beliefs, attitudes, and behaviors. This chapter then ends with recommendations for shifting media messages to showcase more humanizing, and non-stigmatizing, portrayals of people with OUDs. In focusing on people with OUDs, the chapter does not consider portrayals of chronic pain and chronic pain patients who have prescriptions for opioids; for this discussion, see Chap. 5.

3.2 Stigmatizing Language and Media Portrayals

This chapter analyzes media portrayals of the opioid crisis through the lens of stigma communication. Stigma has been defined as both "an attribute that is deeply discrediting" (Goffman 1963, 3) as well as a process through which five interrelated subprocesses converge—that of stereotyping, labeling, distinguishing "us" versus "them," status loss, and discrimination (Link and Phelan 2001). These definitions generally concern public stigma, or the stigmatized beliefs, attitudes, and behaviors exhibited by "normal" society toward a societally stigmatized group. According to the model of stigma communication (MSC), public stigma gets communicated and circulated through four types of messages: *marks* that affix a stigmatizing cue, often disgust-evoking, to the stigmatized person (e.g., dirty needles, images of unkempt people); *labels* that reduce a stigmatized person to their stigmatized group identity (e.g., "addict" rather than "person with an OUD"); *responsibility/etiology* messages that communicate choice for the stigma condition and control over ridding oneself of it (e.g., "people chose to use drugs"); and *peril messages* that signal the stigmatized group poses some harm to others (e.g., the sentiment that people with OUDs are morally and/or physically dangerous; Smith 2007; Ledford 2025). Revisiting the opioid incident from this chapter's introduction, for example, the word "addict" was a stigma label whereas language like "unscarred vein" and "surrounded by syringes" were stigma marks. As will be discussed throughout this chapter, stigma labels, marks, responsibility, and peril have all been linked to harmful stigmatizing beliefs, attitudes, and behaviors (Kelly and Westerhoff 2010; Goodyear et al. 2018; Ledford et al. 2022; Ledford, 2025).

In talking about stigmatizing language in opioid-related media content, it is necessary to also consider how we as researchers write about opioids. Experts generally recommend avoiding language like "substance/opioid abuse" given the way these terms have been used to blame (and thus insinuate a responsibility message, per Smith 2007) people with OUDs for their disorders. Research also suggests avoiding stigmatizing *labels* like "addict" and "junkie" given the stigmatizing attitudes these words have cultivated (Kelly and Westerhoff 2010; Goodyear et al. 2018;

Ledford et al. 2022). This chapter thus adopts the language of "people with OUDs" in recognition that this term removes stigma labeling and responsibility messages. The chapter also intentionally uses the term "opioid crisis" as opposed to "opioid epidemic" given the rhetorical association between epidemic and disease and the potential stigmatizing consequences of that association. Although it is challenging to choose any term that removes normative, and thus potentially stigmatizing, expectations in talking about the opioid crisis (Buchman et al. 2017), this author hopes that, at minimum, the discussion of these choices prompts more thoughtful choices among those reading and utilizing this chapter for stigma-reduction.

The following sections of this chapter will review and analyze how news, entertainment, and social media portray the opioid crisis, with a particular focus on how these portrayals present more or less stigmatizing representations.

3.3 News Media Portrayals

Given that news media reporting of the opioid crisis has increased in tandem with rising opioid overdose deaths (Hswen et al. 2020), it is no wonder that scholars have devoted attention to the content and impacts of opioid-related news coverage. Some of them have analyzed how news media portray the U.S. opioid crisis, focusing on both written news media content (McGinty et al. 2016; McGinty et al. 2019a; McGinty et al. 2019b; Bessette et al. 2022) as well as images and visuals used in news reporting (Scott 2021; Welhausen 2023). Their research suggests that news coverage of the opioid crisis is still rife with stigmatizing portrayals, particularly those that utilize stigma labels and situate the crisis within a criminal justice perspective. For example, several content analyses have revealed that news stories tend to focus on crimes people with OUDs commit and the role of law enforcement in stopping these crimes (McGinty et al. 2016; Willis and Painter 2019; Scott 2021). The focus on criminality in news reporting serves a stigmatizing function by framing the opioid crisis as a criminal justice issue and people with OUDs as criminals in need of jail time. Other research illustrates that news stories still circulate stigmatizing labels like "addict" and "abuser" despite the 2017 updated Associated Press (AP) guidelines to remove these terms (McGinty et al. 2019a; Bessette et al. 2022). Although there have been more humanizing portrayals of opioids over time, particularly of white people with OUDs

(McLean 2017), as well as more solution-focused reporting (McGinty et al. 2019b; Russell et al. 2019), much news coverage of the opioid crisis still endorses stigmatizing portrayals of people with OUDs.

In addition to analyzing the content of news reports, several studies have revealed the harmful outcomes of stigmatizing news stories about people with OUDs (Ledford 2025; Ledford et al. 2022). For example, experimental research has found that stigmatizing labels (e.g., "addict," "abuser") harm people's feelings, attitudes, and behaviors toward people with OUDs (Goodyear et al. 2018; Ledford et al. 2022). One of the most concerning behavioral outcomes from the opioid stigma research is policy-support, as people who endorse stigma toward people with OUDs are more likely to support punitive policies like jail time over treatment-oriented policies such as rehabilitation (Kennedy-Hendricks et al. 2017). Furthermore, peril messages that mention the social, physical, or emotional harms people with OUDs cause to those around them have directly dampened support for Narcan and rehabilitation policies (Ledford 2025) and prompted negative emotions, avoidance, and the desire to isolate people with OUDs from society (Sattler et al. 2021).

3.3.1 Stories Told About People with OUDs

One of the major ways that stigmatizing news stories talk about people with OUDs is by suggesting that the opioid crisis is a criminal justice issue. Analyzing a national sample of 673 print and television news stories about opioids from 1998 to 2012, McGinty et al. (2016) found that during that time, newspapers still largely framed the opioid crisis as a criminal justice issue. This appeared in two ways: illegal drug dealing was the most mentioned cause of the opioid crisis in the sampled articles that mentioned a cause, and among articles mentioning a solution, arresting and prosecuting drug dealers was the most common fix. By mentioning a specific cause of the crisis, these stories attributed responsibility to people who sell and use opioids illegally. Responsibility/etiology messages are one of the four types of stigma messages Smith (2007) highlights, as these messages serve to put blame for a stigma condition on a group of people and thus justify their social isolation (jail time) and exclusion. Other scholars have found this same theme in opioid-related news coverage, including visual depictions of criminal opioid use within *TIME's* "Opioid Diary" (Scott 2021) as well as the *Cincinnati Enquirer's* coverage of opioids from 2015 to 2017, which often focused on crime and law enforcement (Willis and

Painter 2019). In the *Cincinnati Enquirer*, crime-focused stories often used episodic framing, a type of news frame that tells stories in concrete, individual bursts and thus often fails to acknowledge the nuance or larger contexts of social problems (Willis and Painter 2019). This type of framing can contribute to stigmatizing portrayals of people with OUDs through its reductive presentation of the opioid crisis, which does not acknowledge other responsible actors for the crisis (e.g., the government and pharmaceutical companies).

News outlets seem to also be responsible for circulating stigmatizing labels like "addict" and "abuser." One study found that nearly *half* of 6399 sampled national news articles from 2008 to 2018 mentioned a stigmatizing term related to opioids and that articles published between 2017 and 2018 used more stigmatizing language compared to coverage a decade earlier (McGinty et al. 2019a). Even though the AP updated its guidelines in 2017 to prohibit the use of these terms, national news outlets like *USA Today, Los Angeles Times,* and *New York Times* still utilize stigmatizing labels in their reporting (Bessette et al. 2022). In Bessette et al.'s (2022) analysis, only *New York Times* articles included significantly fewer stigmatizing terms after the AP update.

However, due to the impacts of the opioid crisis on white Americans, opioid-related news coverage has begun to humanize people with OUDs, especially white people with OUDs. Historically, news media often portrayed people who used crack cocaine as poor Black people (e.g., Cobbina 2008). The opioid crisis, on the other hand, disproportionately affected white people in its early stage and was depicted as a "white problem," which led to more humanizing portrayals of people with OUDs (McLean 2017). For example, a study analyzing Utah's coverage of the opioid crisis in 2015 and 2016 found that "while only a few stories made explicit mention of race, the news coverage implicitly focused on the idea that the opioid epidemic affects middle-class white people" (Richards 2018, 22). Moreover, thematically analyzing Pittsburgh news coverage related to three surges in heroin overdoses, McLean (2017) found that, over time, local newspapers dedicated increasingly more space to profiling people with heroin OUDs who were white and portrayed these individuals as more victimized than the earlier accounts of urban Black people.

News stories have also increasingly begun to explore public health and policy solutions to the opioid crisis, shifting from framing the crisis as a criminal justice problem to treating it as a public health issue. Of a sample of 2016–2017 Ohio newspaper posts on Facebook, nearly one-third emphasized the importance of a public health approach and legislation to tackle the opioid crisis (Russell et al. 2019). Although another nearly one-third of articles still adopted the law enforcement frame found in past research, the shift toward a focus on public health and policy solutions may represent a turning point in news media reporting. Analyzing national opioid-related coverage from 2013 to 2017, another study found that the number of stories mentioning a public health and/or policy solution to the opioid crisis consistently increased during that time (McGinty et al. 2019b). In addition, the mention of criminal justice solutions decreased over time.

3.3.2 Stories Told by People with OUDs

Many of the stories told about people with OUDs in news media often present these stories from a third-person perspective. The third-person perspective makes sense from a journalistic lens: journalists interview potential contributors, highlight the quotes that make the story, and use their skills as trained journalists to present the story and weave in first-person quotes from the individuals with OUDs. However, research suggests that first-person stories about people with OUDs are more beneficial for reducing psychological reactance to the stories as well as perceived threat of and desired social distance from people with OUDs (Ma et al. 2023). An added benefit is that first-person stories about opioids can increase identification with the character in the story and promote prevention-oriented attitudes and behaviors among the audience (Cao 2024).

There is unfortunately a dearth of research on the contents of first-person news narratives about people with OUDs. Rather, scholars have studied the influence of first-person stories about OUDs more broadly (Ma et al. 2023; Cao 2024) or have analyzed what themes or story content are effective for stigma reduction (Livingston et al. 2012; Heley et al. 2020). Accordingly, much more research should be conducted to analyze how stories are told *by* people with OUDs in news media, especially since these stories have been found to serve a de-stigmatizing function.

3.4 Entertainment Media Portrayals

Entertainment media represent a wide range of media sources designed to entertain audiences. This chapter focuses on television and film in discussing entertainment media given the prevalence of storytelling about the opioids crisis and people with OUDs through these media sources, particularly within the last decade. Popular television shows like ABC's *Grey's Anatomy* and its related spinoff *Private Practice*, HBO's *Euphoria*, and Fox's *House* provide detailed, fictional accounts of main characters who struggle with OUDs. Meanwhile, Netflix's *Painkiller* and Hulu's *Dopesick* both present dramatized accounts of the origins of the U.S. opioid crisis based on the real story of Purdue Pharma and the Sackler family. Documentary filmmakers have also sought to contribute to on-screen dialogue about the crisis. *Recovery Boys* tells the stories of four men navigating OUD recovery in the state of West Virginia, offering one of the few mediated and nonfictional depictions from the perspective of people with OUDs. West Virginia is also the setting of the short documentary film, *Heroin(e)*, an accounting of the women—including local fire chief Jan Rader of Huntington, West Virginia—working to mitigate the deadly impact of the opioid crisis. Taking a starkly different approach to storytelling, comedian John Mulaney also released a Netflix comedy special, *Baby J*, in 2023, of which the central focus is his navigation of addiction and recovery. All released in the twenty-first century, these documentaries, shows, and films illustrate the significant attention dedicated to opioid-related topics by the entertainment industry.

Entertainment media's portrayals of the opioid crisis and people with OUDs are widely understudied, but the limited existing research offers some insights into these portrayals as well as their effects on viewers. For example, *Dopesick* has been critiqued for its simplistic representation of the opioid crisis, with scholars arguing that while it can be commended for evoking sympathy toward people with OUDs and attributing responsibility to Purdue Pharma, the series ultimately portrays OUDs as solely a problem rather than as a problem with a clear solution outside of legal consequences for Purdue Pharma (Piqué-Buisan et al. 2024). *House MD* has also been critiqued for the way it stigmatized the main character as aggressive, dishonest, and drug-seeking because of his Vicodin misuse and clinical depression diagnosis (Biddy 2018). Even though *Euphoria's* representation of drug use was critiqued by the Drug Abuse Resistance Education program (D.A.R.E.) for glamorizing drug use (Rosenblatt

2022), an empirical study recently found that the show served a de-stigmatizing purpose for Gen Z (Gierzynski et al. 2024). Using an online experiment, the authors found that compared to those who were not primed to actively think about the show, participants who were primed to remember the main characters of *Euphoria* expressed more empathy toward people who use drugs, more attributions to external factors causing addiction, and more support for treatment and harm reduction policies.

This limited evidence suggests a need for more research analyzing the entertainment media portrayals of opioid use. It is important to study such portrayals because of the affordances that entertainment media offer. Specifically, entertainment programs usually have more time and space for nuanced storylines, as the characters of television shows often live in the realities of their viewers for months, years, or even decades in the case of *Grey's Anatomy*.

3.4.1 Stories Told About People with OUDs

3.4.1.1 Nonfiction Stories

Many entertainment sources that provide nonfiction accounts of the experiences of people with OUDs do not tell these people's stories from their point of view. Rather, these accounts, including those in *Painkiller, Dopesick,* and *Heroin(e),* tell the stories of individuals with OUDs primarily through the lens of someone else. For example, *Painkiller* primarily provides first-person observations from the perspectives of a lawyer suing Purdue Pharma as well as parents who open each episode discussing their child who died from an opioid overdose. In the documentary *Heroin(e),* the primary storyteller is Jan Rader, the fire chief in Huntington, West Virginia, during the time of the documentary being produced. Given the documentary style of *Heroin(e),* taking a further look into its portrayal offers useful insight into nonfiction depictions of the opioid crisis by entertainment media.

A documentary dedicated to the heroines of the opioid crisis in Huntington, West Virginia, *Heroine(e)* attempts to showcase the "reality" of the opioid crisis but may also perpetuate stigma toward people with OUDs. At the beginning of the documentary, Chief Rader attributes the opioid crisis to a range of systemic factors, commenting on how "hopelessness, unemployment and lack of education" work together to create a "recipe of disaster" resulting in a tremendous loss of life from opioid overdoses. She also reflects on the fact that "West Virginia is mainly a blue-collar state" so it has "a lot of people that work hard for a living, do a lot of physical labor. There's a lot of injuries, lot of people in this area got hooked on pills through a legitimate injury, and uh, have now moved on to heroin because they can't get pills anymore." This acknowledgment of systemic factors contributing to the opioid crisis is a positive step toward de-stigmatizing people with OUDs. The documentary continues its storytelling from the perspectives of the community advocates, especially women, supporting people with OUDs, including Chief Jan Rader, a drug court judge, and a woman who volunteers to help sex workers with OUDs seek rehabilitation. No doubt, these women have helped the people of Huntington, West Virginia. However, depicting these women as saviors of people with OUDs, the documentary also, and perhaps inadvertently, portrays people with OUDs as low-power individuals in need of help, being dragged out of a room where they have overdosed, and being chastised by a drug court judge. *Heroin(e)* thus does represent some aspects of the reality of the opioid crisis and brings public attention to its gravity, but in doing so also in part denies the agency and humanity of people with OUDs in favor of a hero-centric storyline.

3.4.1.2 Fiction Stories

The prominent fictional accounts of people with OUDs in television shows shed light on the ways that people without OUDs talk about the disorder. *Grey's Anatomy* is a useful case to analyze given that one of the main characters, Dr. Amelia Shepherd, of the show is in recovery from an OUD during the series. The drama walks viewers through the personal and professional lives of surgical residents at a hospital in Seattle, Washington. In Amelia's storyline, there are instances where people question her judgment and character, illustrating the common stigmatizing perception that people with OUDs are untrustworthy. Amelia's first entrance in *Grey's Anatomy* in Season 7, Episode 3 demonstrates this when her own brother and fellow neurosurgeon, Dr. Derek Shepherd, questions her surgical judgment. When his wife, Meredith, expresses confusion about Derek's hostility toward Amelia, Derek asks Meredith: "When you totaled your mother's car, were you high on pain pills?...Did you steal your brother's prescription pad so you could feed your addiction?" Upon seeing Meredith's surprise, Derek continues: "and then when she went home, she OD-ed. She was dead for three minutes. I saved her. That's what she put my mother through after losing my father and raising five kids on her own. So no, I don't trust her in my OR [operating room], okay?" As the first depiction of someone with an OUD in the show, this episode, viewed in isolation, could contribute to stigmatizing perceptions of people with OUDs; it is only through the subsequent episodes that the writers give Amelia's storyline more nuance, complexity, and humanity (discussed later in the chapter).

Amelia's storyline stands in contrast to the mass opioid overdose incident faced by the doctors of *Grey's Anatomy* in Season 15, Episode 14. Three minutes into the episode, two doctors are almost hit when a car comes speeding through the ambulance bay, slows down, a passenger pushes an unconscious person out of the car, and the driver speeds away. The doctors recognize the signs of an overdose and immediately note: "Pinpoint pupils. Get some Narcan, a crash cart, and some O2 [oxygen]. I think we got an OD." More patients enter the emergency room shortly after; all of them are given multiple doses of Narcan. The majority of people overdosed seem to be teenagers, including one teenager whom Amelia had taken under her wing to mentor and support through recovery. While the show tries to showcase the support network of the people affected by the opioid crisis, it also reinforces dominant stigma toward people with OUDs. A surgeon remarks at the end of a surgery: "she's all good, and with no hands to shoot up for the next three months, hopefully she'll actually manage to detox." Even a homeless man who was in the park during the overdose incident remarks: "I'm not like them. They're bringing down the neighborhood if you ask me."

These storylines demonstrate the challenge faced by a third-person approach to humanizing opioid-related storytelling and point toward the need for more complex and nuanced, first-person approaches to talking about opioids in entertainment media.

3.4.2 Stories Told by People with OUDs

3.4.2.1 Nonfiction Stories

More entertainment programs have begun to dedicate space to sharing the experiences of people with OUDs primarily from their perspective. Netflix's documentary *Recovery Boys* and John Mulaney's comedy special *Baby J* represent two of the major accounts in this aim. Since *Recovery Boys* is one of the few documentary depictions from the perspective of people in recovery, this section further analyzes its portrayals of people with OUDs.

Recovery Boys centers on the experiences of four men navigating their experiences with opioid use and recovery. The documentary opens with narration from one of the four men: "I came home one day, and my wife was using heroin. I fell in love with it pretty quick." Contrary to the way many entertainment programs begin by showing graphic depictions of opioid use and overdose, *Recovery Boys* opens with first-person narration and offers humanizing portrayals of people with OUDs. It depicts the men's lives in Jacob's Ladder, a farm-based rehabilitation center in West Virginia, showing them smiling and laughing with one another, expressing excitement to work on the farm, and even doing yoga together. They are also portrayed as people with families. Early in the film, one of the characters uses photographs to introduce his family to viewers, telling complex stories of addiction within his family and showing a photo of his child.

In contrast to *Dopesick* and *Painkiller's* focus on the pharmaceutical industry as the primary entity responsible for the rise of OUDs in the U.S., *Recovery boys* highlights the importance of acceptance of individual responsibility, which represents a key tenet of recovery for people with OUDs and a principle of the commonly used recovery program, Narcotics Anonymous (G. Chen 2022). The documentary does acknowledge a more nuanced view of responsibility as well, subtly recognizing the role of the social environment (e.g., substance use within families) in the opioid crisis. It also explicitly discusses the role of stigma, as one of the four men reflects: "I read this one book that said the word 'stigma' comes from Greek, and they used to brand people on the face for being a certain caste that was looked down upon by society. And when you're a drug addict, I mean like you dress in a certain way, you look a certain way, I mean the tattoos everything like that, and people take one look at you and judge you. So I can see why people would want to change that perception. Might be something I want to work on in the future. Right now, I do just want to focus on the inside stuff, you know?" This sentiment encapsulates the ethos of the documentary as it depicts the men in recovery as reflexive individuals capable of being aware of and maybe even changing the social structures around them.

3.4.2.2 Fiction Stories

Two of the most prominent fictional accounts of the experiences of people with OUDs from a first-person perspective are in *Grey's Anatomy* and *Euphoria*. Airing in 2005 on the American Broadcasting Company (ABC), *Grey's Anatomy* was recently renewed for its 21st season, making it the network's longest running primetime drama (Otterson 2018). In Season 7, viewers meet Dr. Amelia Shepherd, who appears again in the next few seasons until becoming a series regular in Season 11. Her storyline as a neurosurgeon navigating recovery from an OUD was the first in the show to shed light on the opioid crisis. *Euphoria*, on the other hand, centers on the experience of the main character Rue Bennet, a 17-year-old navigating her OUD. Produced by the Home Box Office (HBO) company, *Euphoria's* first season aired in 2019, and the show recently began filming for its third season at the start of 2025. In its second season, *Euphoria* was HBO's second-most-watched show, lagging only behind Game of Thrones (Maas 2022). Although the critical acclaim of both these television shows has led to public dialogue about how they represent the opioid crisis (MacCarthy and Stein 2019; McMullan 2022), few scholars have empirically examined the way these shows portray opioids and the resulting impacts with only one notable exception of the previously cited study showing that *Euphoria* prompted de-stigmatizing beliefs and attitudes among Gen Z participants (Gierzynski et al. 2024). Since *Grey's Anatomy's* portrayals of opioid use have not been systematically explored thus far, this chapter analyzes several of its portrayals as a case study for portrayals of opioid use by entertainment media.

The primary portrayals of opioids in *Grey's Anatomy* and its spinoff *Private Practice* follow the life of neurosurgeon Dr. Amelia Shepherd, who enters both shows in recovery from an OUD. In the fifth season of *Private Practice*, Amelia relapses after the traumatic death by suicide of a friend. The show depicts the aftermath of her relapse: a drug-induced romantic relationship, problems at work and with her friends, and a run-in with the police. Amelia's relapse culminates during Season 5, Episode 8 when the doctors at her practice stage an ultimately ineffective intervention. It is not until the end of the episode, when Amelia wakes to find her new boyfriend, Ryan, dead from an opioid overdose, that Amelia acknowledges she is ready for rehab. Later, when Amelia enters *Grey's Anatomy* as a series regular, she navigates the challenges of sobriety and recovery, with a relapse from alcohol in Season 12. However, the show largely portrays her as coping with stress through the healthy expression of emotion rather than through drugs or alcohol. Though she faces challenges in how others see her when they find out about her drug use, Amelia's story itself is one of ultimate recovery and hope.

The entertainment media examples discussed here seem to represent more complexity and humanity in their portrayals of the opioid crisis compared to news media's depictions. This is likely in part due to the format of television and film: as opposed to short, palatable news stories consumed quickly, shows and movies can showcase greater character development and storylines over a longer period and through a multimedia format.

3.5 Social Media

Social media has become a major interest in many academic fields, and an increasing number of studies have begun to track how people are talking about opioids on social media platforms. Several of these studies use a geolocation framework to see if the number of opioid overdoses in a specific location corresponds to the social media discourse about opioids in that same location (Sarker et al. 2019; Black et al. 2020; Flores and Young 2021). These studies have begun making the case that public health researchers can track social media discourse to identify and subsequently prevent rising opioid overdoses. Other social media researchers have analyzed the content of comments and posts about opioids on platforms such as reddit, Twitter/X, and YouTube (Chan et al. 2015; Chancellor et al. 2019; Jain et al. 2020; Ittefaq et al. 2023; O'Kelly et al. 2024). Reddit, in particular, may offer people with OUDs a safe and supportive space to talk about their disorder and their experiences with recovery (D'Agostino et al. 2017; Chancellor et al. 2019).

Responses to social media content about opioids are limited but preliminarily suggest that people seem to interact more with media-rich posts, posts from media sources, and risk-based messages. Jain et al. (2020) found that people were more likely to retweet posts that included both videos and text compared to text-only posts, tweets originating from media sources and personalities compared to those from health organizations, and tweets mentioning disease-related information such as the causes, impact, and treatment related to opioids. O'Kelly et al. (2024) similarly found that YouTube videos created by non-medical sources like independent users, media organizations (e.g., talk shows, radio shows, and news organizations), and television series received more views and likes compared to videos produced by medical organizations. Meanwhile, Ittefaq et al. (2023) found that most YouTube comments in response to John Oliver's opioid-focused *Last Week Tonight* episodes were about the side effects of opioid use.

3.5.1 Stories Told About People with OUDs

Much of the social media research about opioid-related content has focused on how people talk about opioids on Twitter/X. In their analysis of opioid-related tweets in March and April 2014, one study found that three-fifths of tweets discussed general thoughts and perceptions about opioid use, varying in their mention of positive (e.g., "Hydros fix everything") or negative perceptions (e.g., "I don't understand the culture of young people who think its okay to pop Molly's, Percocet, Oxycotin, Xanax, etc.") or the people who misused opioids (Chan et al. 2015, 6). Along the same lines, another Twitter/X-focused study that explored tweets in October and November 2018 found that the discussion of opioids rarely focused on specific stories within the crisis (Jain et al. 2020). Rather, people discussed opioids in varying ways. Some talked about who was responsible for the crisis; others focused on the harms caused by and the solutions to addiction; and still others mentioned the number of deaths from opioid overdose (Jain et al. 2020). Analyzing how health professionals talk about opioids on Twitter/X, another study found that between 2009 and 2021, health professionals were less likely than non-health professionals to use stigmatizing terms to talk about addiction; health professionals were more aware of the stigmatizing terms to avoid in talking about opioids and used less of stigmatizing terms like "abuse" and "addict" compared to Twitter users who were not health professionals (Scott Graham et al. 2022).

A few other studies have analyzed opioid-related posts/videos and comments on YouTube and Facebook. One study sought to examine what type of YouTube content exists related to OUD treatment (O'Kelly et al. 2024). It found that, among 70 relevant videos, just over one-fifth presented quality information about OUD treatment options. More concerning was that the videos with higher quality information had fewer views "despite YouTube's default setting to present credible content from verified health sources at the top of each results page" (O'Kelly et al. 2024, 5). When responding to Ohio news organization's posts, Facebook users most often made emotional comments, many of which expressed stigmatizing emotions such as fear and embarrassment of living in a place with high rates of opioid use (Russell et al. 2019). Choice and responsibility were the second most common focus of the responses to the posts by Ohio newspapers, with people emphasizing the role of individuals with OUDs in their addiction. Such individual responsibility messages imply that a person's stigmatizing attribute is completely within their control (Smith 2007). One person even explicitly wrote: "At what point, if ever, do you take responsibility for taking something that you know will kill you?" (Russell et al. 2019, 706).

3.5.2 Stories Told by People with OUDs

Reddit has emerged as a space used by people with OUDs to talk about their experiences and recovery (D'Agostino et al. 2017; Chancellor et al. 2019). In an analysis of 100 reddit posts within an opioid-related self-help group, D'Agostino et al. (2017) found that most of the posts and related comments focused on either seeking or giving help. Posts in this group often discussed the harm that opioid use caused to people's lives and relationships, and comments often centered around sharing personal experiences. As the authors argue, these posts carved out an authentic space for reddit users, affording them safety, vis-à-vis anonymity, to openly share their journey with opioid misuse and/or recovery and seek non-judgmental social support. Another study analyzed 1.44 million posts across 63 subreddits to identify which alternative treatments (i.e., non-medically approved or supervised methods) people with OUDs seek for managing their opioid withdrawal and recovery (Chancellor et al. 2019). Of the recovery-focused posts, several endorsed the use of non-approved medications for opioid treatment, including benzodiazepines like Xanax, which can interact with opioids to raise the risk of overdose, as well as kratom, an herbal supplement people have reported using to manage opioid withdrawal because of its stimulant properties that mirror opioid effects (National Institute on Drug Abuse 2022). Although not currently FDA-approved, researchers have begun to investigate whether kratom's treatment potential outweighs its adverse effects (Johns Hopkins Medicine 2020).

People with OUDs have also shared their personal experiences on Twitter/X, though with less depth than on reddit. Some of these tweets discuss experiences with recovery. For example, one tweeter stated: "After taking #opioids daily for pain for 12+ years; I'm on day 4 of no pain pills or muscle relaxers. Thank you #weed!" (Jain et al. 2020, 77). However, one study found that most tweets discussing personal experiences focused on the experience of engaging in opioid misuse, including people joking or making casual references about opioid use (e.g., "Vicodin and vodka get me in my drake like a champ"; Chan et al. 2015, 5).

Overall, the studies reviewed here suggest that reddit provides a non-stigmatizing space to talk openly about opioids recovery with other people and that Twitter/X is not a prominent medium used for community-building and support-seeking by people with OUDs.

3.6 Recommendations for Changing Media Messages

Stigma reduction research generally suggests three primary strategies for reducing stigma: education, contact, and protest (Committee on the Science of Changing Behavioral Health Social Norms et al. 2016). Educational strategies focus on increasing awareness of the stigmatized issue and correcting misinformation to reduce the negative beliefs and attitudes about people who are stigmatized. Contact helps people reduce stigma by exposing them to real people with the stigmatized condition, showcasing those individuals' humanity rather than only their stigmatized condition. Contact also includes mediated contact, the type evidenced in many of the cases analyzed in this chapter, wherein people are exposed to those with stigmatized conditions through mediated representations. Finally, protests are used to advocate for better representations of people with stigmatized conditions as well as more justice and support for these people. Although evidence is limited on the medium- and long-term effects of these stigma reduction strategies, researchers have found that contact-based strategies and positive storytelling about people with OUDs generally reduce substance use stigma more than education-only strategies (Livingston et al. 2012; Judd et al. 2023).

Given that news stories are often read in isolation at one point in time, removing stigmatizing language and stigmatizing stories is especially crucial for journalists. Journalists should ensure that they follow the AP's guidelines to avoid stigmatizing *labels* like "addict," "abuser," and "junkie" that promote and/or reinforce stigma (Kelly and Westerhoff 2010; Ashford et al. 2018; Ledford et al. 2022) and replace the labels with first-person descriptions like "people with OUDs." Removing stigmatizing terminology must also include the removal of stigmatizing *marks*. Rather than describing or showcasing stigmatizing images of people with OUDs being arrested, appearing unkempt, or in the same image as needles or drugs, journalists should use more humanizing language and images (e.g., pictures of people with OUDs smiling, living the rest of their lives, and/or interacting with their social support networks). To remove *peril* messages, journalists should avoid focusing on the physical, social, or moral harm that people with OUDs cause to others since these messages prompt stigmatizing attitudes and behaviors (Sattler et al. 2021; Ledford 2025). Instead, they should recount positive stories of recovery and hope (Livingston et al. 2012). Finally, to remove the focus on individual *responsibility* for opioids, journalists should acknowledge the complexity and nuance of the causes of the opioid crisis in their reporting, which may be best accomplished through narrative storytelling. Rather than blaming either Purdue Pharma or people with OUDs exclusively, journalists can explain how a person's choices are affected by larger systemic factors (e.g., social determinants of health) and societal trends (e.g., the prevalence of the experience in a society). These stories should also explore solutions, as research has suggested that a discussion of nuanced responsibility along with a policy solution to the opioid crisis can successfully reduce opioid stigma (Heley et al. 2020). Focusing on treatment-oriented solutions to the opioid crisis can also shift the focus away from a criminal/law enforcement framing of the crisis.

As for entertainment media agents such as writers and producers, a key takeaway is to tell nuanced first-person narratives that highlight the authenticity and humanity of people with OUDs. Entertainment media usually offer longer-form content, allowing viewers to be transported through films, documentaries (e.g., *Recovery Boys*), and television series (e.g., *Euphoria*), which makes these genres particularly conducive to reducing stigma through humanizing and positive stories from the viewpoints of people with OUDs. Of course, these programs should also work to remove stigmatizing language and portrayals as noted above.

Finally, social media content presents a challenge for a sweeping stigma reduction recommendation, as the agent of change is the individual—the person creating and/or sharing the social media content. Currently, it seems that there is not enough accurate information about opioids treatment on social media (O'Kelly et al. 2024). Furthermore, people on social media tend to engage more with media personalities and organizations rather than health organizations (Jain et al. 2020; O'Kelly et al. 2024). As such, any media organization or personality who shares opioid-related content should take seriously the call to present accurate and humanizing information. While all individuals should consider their posting habits within this broader context, media organizations face an additional responsibility given the current research findings. Removing stigma label, mark, responsibility, and peril messages is certainly a step in the right direction, as is sharing positive narratives about people with OUDs (Livingston et al. 2012).

To reduce stigmatizing portrayals by the media, journalists, writers, producers, and social media users should consider the research and recommendations explored in this chapter and summarized in Table 3.1.

Table 3.1 Strategies for creating humanizing media portrayals of the opioid crisis

Strategy	*Avoid*	*Use*	*Supporting evidence*
Remove stigma labels	Terms like: "addict" "user" "junkie" "abuser" "abuse" "misuser"	First-person terminology like "person with an opioid use disorder"	(Ashford et al. 2018; Kelly and Westerhoff 2010; Ledford et al. 2022)
Remove stigma marks	Language and images that portray people as dirty, unclean, or unkempt; language and images providing graphics of active drug use like needle injection and snorting pills	Language and images that show people as fully human, living their lives, smiling and in recovery, surrounded by social support	(Scott 2021; Ledford et al. 2022)
Provide nuanced responsibility narratives	Simplistic representations of responsibility, an over-focus on individual responsibility, an exclusive focus on a single factor as responsible	Nuanced storytelling to portray people as making choices embedded within social determinants of health, systemic factors, and a broader social context that shape and constrain their choices	(Heley et al. 2020; Piqué-Buisan et al. 2024)
Remove peril messages	Portraying the social, physical, or moral harms and dangers people with OUDs cause to others	Positive stories of hope and recovery	(Livingston et al. 2012; Sattler et al. 2021; Ledford 2025)
Tell authentic and honest stories about people with OUDs	Third-person stories that utilize stigma messaging and stigmatizing portrayals	Nuanced first-person stories either from the lives of real people or based on the lives of real people	(Ma et al. 2023; Gierzynski et al. 2024)
Focus on treatment-oriented, public health policy solutions	An exclusive focus on the problem without a focus on solutions; emphasizing only individual solutions (e.g., behavior change); Emphasizing criminal justice responses to the opioid crisis	Focus on a public health approach to the opioid crisis, including various treatment options and policies that can make treatment options available	(Kennedy-Hendricks et al. 2017; Heley et al. 2020)

3.7 Conclusion

News, entertainment, and social media play key roles in shaping public understanding of the opioid crisis. Although each platform has unique structures and affordances, the solutions to reducing stigma across these platforms remain the same: remove stigmatizing language and portrayals and focus on humanizing, authentic narratives that showcase people with OUDs as *people* first. Changing how media talk about the opioid crisis will require a great deal of time, energy, and effort. Understanding how the media have been portraying (and stigmatizing) people negatively affected by the opioid crisis and what can be done to de-stigmatize and even humanize these people is only the first step.

References

Ashford, Robert D., Austin M. Brown, and Brenda Curtis. 2018. Substance Use, Recovery, and Linguistics: The Impact of Word Choice on Explicit and Implicit Bias. *Drug and Alcohol Dependence* 189 (August): 131–138. https://doi.org/10.1016/j.drugalcdep.2018.05.005.

Bessette, Lily G., Sacha C. Hauc, Heidi Danckers, Agata Atayde, and Richard Saitz. 2022. The Associated Press Stylebook Changes and the Use of Addiction-Related Stigmatizing Terms in News Media. *Substance Abuse* 43 (1): 127–130. https://doi.org/10.1080/08897077.2020.1748167.

Biddy, Kacey J. 2018. Mental Illness and the Primetime Medical Drama: Representation in Grey's Anatomy and House M.D. Master's thesis, Middle Tennessee State University. ProQuest (10789692).

Black, Joshua C., Zachary R. Margolin, Richard A. Olson, and Richard C. Dart. 2020. Online Conversation Monitoring to Understand the Opioid Epidemic: Epidemiological Surveillance Study. *JMIR Public Health and Surveillance* 6 (2): e17073. https://doi.org/10.2196/17073.

Buchman, Daniel Z., Pamela Leece, and Aaron Orkin. 2017. The Epidemic as Stigma: The Bioethics of Opioids. *Journal of Law, Medicine & Ethics* 45 (4): 607–620. https://doi.org/10.1177/1073110517750600.

Cao, Xiaoxia. 2024. The Impacts of Narrative Perspectives of Anti-Prescription Opioid Campaigns: The Mediating Roles of Identification, Perceived Severity, and Anticipated Guilt. *Health Communication* 39 (2): 244–257. https://www.tandfonline.com/doi/full/10.1080/10410236.2022.2163110.

CBS News. 2016. 28 ODs in 4 Hours: How the Heroin Epidemic Choked a W.Va. City. September 4. https://www.cbsnews.com/news/4-hours-in-huntington-va-how-the-heroin-epidemic-choked-a-city/.

CDC. 2021. Opioid Overdose: Understanding the Epidemic. March 17. https://www.cdc.gov/drugoverdose/epidemic/index.html.

CDC. 2025. Provisional Drug Overdose Death Counts. April 7. https://www.cdc.gov/nchs/nvss/vsrr/drug-overdose-data.htm.

Chan, Brian, Andrea Lopez, and Urmimala Sarkar. 2015. The Canary in the Coal Mine Tweets: Social Media Reveals Public Perceptions of Non-Medical Use of Opioids. *PLOS ONE* 10 (8): e0135072. https://doi.org/10.1371/journal.pone.0135072.

Chancellor, Stevie, George Nitzburg, Andrea Hu, Francisco Zampieri, and Munmun De Choudhury. 2019. Discovering Alternative Treatments for Opioid Use Recovery Using Social Media. In *Proceedings of the 2019 CHI Conference on Human Factors in Computing Systems*, 1–15. Glasgow Scotland, UK: ACM. https://doi.org/10.1145/3290605.3300354.

Chen, Gila. 2022. The Role of Acceptance and Change in Recovery from Substance Use Disorders. *Journal of Psychoactive Drugs* 54 (4): 340–347. https://doi.org/10.1080/02791072.2021.1979700.

Chen, Yingxi, Meredith S. Shiels, David Thomas, Neal D. Freedman, Amy Berrington, and de González. 2019. Premature Mortality From Drug Overdoses: A Comparative Analysis of 13 Organisation for Economic Co-Operation and Development Member Countries With High-Quality Death Certificate Data, 2001 to 2015. *Annals of Internal Medicine* 170 (5): 352–354. https://doi.org/10.7326/M18-2415.

Cobbina, Jennifer E. 2008. Race and Class Differences in Print Media Portrayals of Crack Cocaine and Methamphetamine. *Journal of Criminal Justice and Popular Culture* 15 (2): 145–167.

Committee on the Science of Changing Behavioral Health Social Norms; Board on Behavioral, Cognitive, and Sensory Sciences;Division of Behavioral and Social Sciences and Education; National Academies of Sciences, Engineering, and Medicine. 2016. Approaches to Reducing Stigma. In *Ending Discrimination Against People with Mental and Substance Use Disorders: The Evidence for Stigma Change*. Washington (DC): National Academies Press (US). https://www.ncbi.nlm.nih.gov/books/NBK384914/?report=printable.

D'Agostino, Alexandra R., Allison R. Optican, Shaina J. Sowles, Melissa J. Krauss, Kiriam Escobar Lee, and Patricia A. Cavazos-Rehg. 2017. Social Networking Online to Recover from Opioid Use Disorder: A Study of Community Interactions. *Drug and Alcohol Dependence* 181 (December): 5–10. https://doi.org/10.1016/j.drugalcdep.2017.09.010.

Flores, Lidia, and Sean D. Young. 2021. Regional Variation in Discussion of Opioids on Social Media. *Journal of Addictive Diseases* 39 (3): 316–321. https://doi.org/10.1080/10550887.2021.1874804.

Gierzynski, Anthony, Madeleine Blaber, Marjorie Brown, et al. 2024. The 'Euphoria' Effect: A Popular HBO Show, Gen Z, and Drug Policy Beliefs.

Social Science Quarterly 105 (2): 193–210. https://doi.org/10.1111/ssqu.13351.

Goffman, E. 1963. Notes on the Management of Spoiled Identity. Prentice-Hall.

Goodyear, Kimberly, Carolina L. Haass-Koffler, and David Chavanne. 2018. Opioid Use and Stigma: The Role of Gender, Language and Precipitating Events. *Drug and Alcohol Dependence* 185 (April): 339–346. https://doi.org/10.1016/j.drugalcdep.2017.12.037.

Heley, Kathryn, Alene Kennedy-Hendricks, Jeff Niederdeppe, and Colleen L. Barry. 2020. Reducing Health-Related Stigma Through Narrative Messages. *Health Communication* 35 (7): 849–860. https://doi.org/10.1080/10410236.2019.1598614.

Hswen, Yulin, Amanda Zhang, Clark Freifeld, and John S. Brownstein. 2020. Evaluation of Volume of News Reporting and Opioid-Related Deaths in the United States: Comparative Analysis Study of Geographic and Socioeconomic Differences. *Journal of Medical Internet Research* 22 (7): e17693. https://doi.org/10.2196/17693.

Ittefaq, Muhammad, Ali Zain, and Hasnain Bokhari. 2023. Opioids in Satirical News Shows: Exploring Topics, Sentiments, and Engagement in Last Week Tonight on YouTube. *Journal of Health Communication* 28 (1): 53–63. https://doi.org/10.1080/10810730.2023.2176575.

Jain, Parul, Zulfia Zaher, and Imran Mazid. 2020. Opioids on Twitter: A Content Analysis of Conversations Regarding Prescription Drugs on Social Media and Implications for Message Design. *Journal of Health Communication* 25 (1): 74–81. https://doi.org/10.1080/10810730.2019.1707911.

Johns Hopkins Medicine. 2020. Natural Herb Kratom May Have Therapeutic Effects And Relatively Low Potential For Abuse Or Harm, According To A User Survey. February 3. https://www.hopkinsmedicine.org/news/newsroom/news-releases/2020/02/natural-herb-kratom-may-have-therapeutic-effects-and-relatively-low-potential-for-abuse-or-harm-according-to-a-user-survey.

Judd, Hailey, Cristian L. Meier, Ashley C. Yaugher, Emma Campbell, and Kandice Atismé-Bevins. 2023. Opioid Use Disorder Stigma Reduction Through Story Telling Narrative and Sharing: A Qualitative Review and Lessons Learned. *International Journal of Mental Health and Addiction* 21 (1): 468–483. https://doi.org/10.1007/s11469-021-00606-y.

Kelly, John F., and Cassandra M. Westerhoff. 2010. Does it Matter how We Refer to Individuals with Substance-Related Conditions? A Randomized Study of Two Commonly Used Terms. *International Journal of Drug Policy* 21 (3): 202–207. https://doi.org/10.1016/j.drugpo.2009.10.010.

Kennedy-Hendricks, Alene, Colleen L. Barry, Sarah E. Gollust, Margaret E. Ensminger, Margaret S. Chisolm, and Emma E. McGinty. 2017. Social Stigma toward Persons with Prescription Opioid Use Disorder: Associations with Public Support for Punitive and Public Health–Oriented Policies. *Psychiatric Services* 68 (5): 462–469. https://doi.org/10.1176/appi.ps.201600056.

Ledford, Victoria. 2025. The Peril of Opioid Stigma Peril: Experimental Evidence for Removing Danger-Based Health Appeals. *Stigma and Health*. https://doi.org/10.1037/sah0000638.

Ledford, Victoria, Jungkyu Rhys Lim, Kang Namkoong, Junhan Chen, and Yan Qin. 2022. The Influence of Stigmatizing Messages on Danger Appraisal: Examining the Model of Stigma Communication for Opioid-Related Stigma, Policy Support, and Related Outcomes. *Health Communication* 37 (14): 1765–1777. https://doi.org/10.1080/10410236.2021.1920710.

Link, Bruce G., and Jo C. Phelan. 2001. Conceptualizing Stigma. *Annual Review of Sociology* 27:363–385.

Livingston, James D., Teresa Milne, Mei Lan Fang, and Erica Amari. 2012. The Effectiveness of Interventions for Reducing Stigma Related to Substance Use Disorders: A Systematic Review. *Addiction* 107 (1): 39–50. https://doi.org/10.1111/j.1360-0443.2011.03601.x.

Ma, Zexin, Rong Ma, and Victoria Ledford. 2023. Is My Story Better than His Story? Understanding the Effects and Mechanisms of Narrative Point of View in the Opioid Context. *Health Communication* 38 (9): 1847–1855. https://doi.org/10.1080/10410236.2022.2037198.

Maas, Jennifer. 2022. 'Euphoria' Is Now HBO's Second-Most Watched Show Behind 'Game of Thrones.' *Variety* (blog), February 28. https://variety.com/2022/tv/news/euphoria-season-2-finale-ratings-1235192015/.

MacCarthy, Sarah, and Bradley D. Stein. 2019. (Grey's) Anatomy of an Opioid Crisis. https://www.rand.org/pubs/commentary/2019/04/greys-anatomy-of-an-opioid-crisis.html.

McGinty, Emma E., Alene Kennedy-Hendricks, Julia Baller, Jeff Niederdeppe, Sarah Gollust, and Colleen L. Barry. 2016. Criminal Activity or Treatable Health Condition? News Media Framing of Opioid Analgesic Abuse in the United States, 1998–2012. *Psychiatric Services* 67 (4): 405–411. https://doi.org/10.1176/appi.ps.201500065.

McGinty, Emma E., Elizabeth M. Stone, Alene Kennedy-Hendricks, and Colleen L. Barry. 2019a. Stigmatizing Language in News Media Coverage of the Opioid Epidemic: Implications for Public Health. *Preventive Medicine* 124 (July): 110–114. https://doi.org/10.1016/j.ypmed.2019.03.018.

McGinty, Emma E., Elizabeth M. Stone, Alene Kennedy-Hendricks, Kaylynn Sanders, Alexa Beacham, and Colleen L. Barry. 2019b. U.S. News Media Coverage of Solutions to the Opioid Crisis, 2013–2017. *Preventive Medicine* 126 (September): 105771. https://doi.org/10.1016/j.ypmed.2019.105771.

McLean, Katherine. 2017. From 'Junkies' to 'Soccer Moms': Newspaper Representations of Overdose, 1988–2014. *Critical Criminology* 25 (3): 411–432. https://doi.org/10.1007/s10612-017-9350-2.

McMullan, Marie. 2022. What 'Euphoria' Gets Right about Addiction. Vox Magazine, February 17. https://www.voxmagazine.com/arts/tv/what-euphoria-gets-right-about-addiction/article_dedd1856-8dc7-11ec-ac96-d7fa8848b4aa.html.

National Institute on Drug Abuse. 2022. Kratom. National Institutes of Health. March 25. https://nida.nih.gov/research-topics/kratom.

National Institute on Drug Abuse. 2024. Drug Overdose Deaths: Facts and Figures. August 21. https://nida.nih.gov/research-topics/trends-statistics/overdose-death-rates.

O'Kelly, Bridget, Perry Holmes, Anna Cheng, Joshua D. Lee, and Babak Tofighi. 2024. Dissemination of Health Content through Social Networks: YouTube and Opioid Use Disorders. *Journal of Substance Use and Addiction Treatment* 165 (October): 209475. https://doi.org/10.1016/j.josat.2024.209475.

Oldfield, Benjamin J., Jeanette M. Tetrault, and Gretchen Berland. 2021. Addiction Screening—The *A Star Is Born* Movie Series and Destigmatization of Substance Use Disorders. *JAMA* 325 (10): 915. https://doi.org/10.1001/jama.2020.25256.

Otterson, Joe. 2018. 'Grey's Anatomy' Renewed for Season 15 at ABC. *Variety* (blog), April 21. https://variety.com/2018/tv/news/greys-anatomy-renewed-season-15-abc-1202777808/.

Piqué-Buisan, Joel, Josep-E. Baños, and Irene Cambra-Badii. 2024. Telling the Story of the Opioid Crisis: A Narrative Analysis of the TV Series Dopesick. *PLOS ONE* 19 (4): e0301681. https://doi.org/10.1371/journal.pone.0301681.

Richards, Connor. 2018. The Role of Race and Class in Local Media Coverage of Utah's Opioid Epidemic. *The Hinckley Journal of Politics* 18 (1): 18–27.

Rosenblatt, Kalhan. 2022. D.A.R.E. Says HBO's 'Euphoria' Glamorizes Drug Use, Sex and Violence. NBC News, January 26. https://www.nbcnews.com/pop-culture/pop-culture-news/dre-says-hbos-euphoria-glamorizes-drug-use-sex-violence-rcna13631.

Russell, David, Kelly M. Thames, and Naomi J. Spence. 2019. 'It's so Scary How Common this is Now:' Frames in Media Coverage of the Opioid Epidemic by Ohio Newspapers and Themes in Facebook User Reactions. *Information, Communication & Society* 22 (5): 702–708. https://doi.org/10.1080/1369118X.2019.1566393.

Sarker, Abeed, Graciela Gonzalez-Hernandez, Yucheng Ruan, and Jeanmarie Perrone. 2019. Machine Learning and Natural Language Processing for Geolocation-Centric Monitoring and Characterization of Opioid-Related

Social Media Chatter. *JAMA Network Open* 2 (11): e1914672. https://doi.org/10.1001/jamanetworkopen.2019.14672.

Sattler, Sebastian, Farzaneh Zolala, Mohammad Reza Baneshi, Javad Ghasemi, and Saber Amirzadeh Googhari. 2021. Public Stigma Toward Female and Male Opium and Heroin Users. An Experimental Test of Attribution Theory and the Familiarity Hypothesis. *Frontiers in Public Health* 9 (April): https://doi.org/10.3389/fpubh.2021.652876.

Scott, Alex. 2021. Peering Down at the Junkie: Authority and the Visual Construction of Drug Users in *TIME*'s 'Opioid Diary'. *Visual Communication Quarterly* 28 (3): 152–165. https://doi.org/10.1080/15551393.2021.1949721.

Scott Graham, S., Fiona N. Conway, Richard Bottner, and Kasey Claborn. 2022. Opioid Use Stigmatization and Destigmatization in Health Professional Social Media. *Addiction Research & Theory* 30 (5): 375–381. https://doi.org/10.1080/16066359.2022.2061962.

Smith, Rachel A. 2007. Language of the Lost: An Explication of Stigma Communication. *Communication Theory* 17 (4): 462–485. https://doi.org/10.1111/j.1468-2885.2007.00307.x.

Welhausen, Candice A. 2023. Visualizing a Drug Abuse Epidemic: Media Coverage, Opioids, and the Racialized Construction of Public Health Frameworks. *Journal of Technical Writing and Communication* 53 (2): 106–127. https://doi.org/10.1177/00472816221125186.

Willis, Erin, and Chad Painter. 2019. The Needle and the Damage Done: Framing the Heroin Epidemic in the *Cincinnati Enquirer*. *Health Communication* 34 (6): 661–671. https://doi.org/10.1080/10410236.2018.1431023.

CHAPTER 4

Framing the Opioid Crisis: Exploring the Effects of Frames on Perceptions, Stigma, Behavior, Policy, and Intervention Support

Virgil L. Hayes Jr.

4.1 Introduction

The opioid crisis remains one of the most severe public health issues in the United States. In 2022 alone, a record 107,941 individuals died of a drug overdose (Spencer et al. 2023). However, in 2023, public health experts reported a decrease in the number of fatal overdoses as the rate of overdoses dropped from 32.6 per 100,000 in 2022 to 31.3 per 100,000 in 2023 (Garnett and Miniño 2024). While this progress should certainly be celebrated, a closer look at the data shows that the impact of the opioid crisis was heightened among marginalized communities. For example, while the rates of drug overdose declined for White individuals in 2023, rates for other racial groups remained the same and, in some instances, even increased (Garnett and Miniño 2024). Indeed, data shows that for Native Hawaiian and Black communities, overdose rates have steadily increased in recent years. Moreover, there were increases in rates of

V. L. Hayes Jr. (✉)
School of Social Work, University of Missouri, Columbia, MO, USA
e-mail: vlhn3h@mail.missouri.edu

X. Cao (ed.), *Fighting the Opioid Crisis with Communication*,
https://doi.org/10.1007/978-3-032-31162-7_4

overdose among certain age groups (Garnett and Miniño 2024). For example, although rates of fatal overdoses decreased for people between the ages of 15 and 54 in 2023, adults 55 and older experienced an increase in overdose rates. The economic impact of the opioid crisis is equally alarming. According to the Joint Economic Committee (2022), the cost of the opioid epidemic increased by 37% from 2017 to 2020, bringing the estimated total cost of this public health crisis to a staggering over $1.5 trillion per year.

Despite rising public awareness and accumulating evidence supporting the effectiveness of medication-assisted therapy and harm reduction services, these treatment and life-saving measures still face public resistance. This resistance often stems from stigma, misconceptions, and the intentional language used in media and policy discourse (Madden 2019). Drug use and overdose are not solitary issues; they are inseparably linked to broader social, political, and economic factors that dictate risk and access to care. Researchers like Collins et al. (2019) posit that environments characterized by poverty, housing instability, racial disparities, and limited healthcare access elevate the risk of developing substance use disorders (SUDs), such as opioid use disorder, and facing obstacles to recovery.

Communication significantly influences the visibility of these structural determinants to the public and policymakers. This is where research on the framing effect becomes crucial. The language, tone, and context used to portray opioid use disorder and its solutions not only mold public perception but also influence political commitment. The framing effect pertains to how information is presented and how those presentations impact attitudes, beliefs, and behaviors. Regarding the opioid crisis, framing can dictate whether the public perceives the opioid epidemic as a criminal justice matter or a public health crisis, whether people who use drugs are seen as criminal offenders or individuals in need of empathy, and whether life-saving measures are viewed as enablers of drug use or viable recovery options.

Research in health communication defines framing as the presentation of information in a way that highlights certain aspects of an issue to influence perception and attitude (Guenther et al. 2021). The chapter provides an overview of empirical findings from framing effect research within the context of the opioid crisis, analyzing how different framing strategies can alter perspectives among the public, policymakers, law enforcement, and White Americans. It also examines how framing interacts with factors such as race and community context in shaping attitudes and behaviors.

Additionally, the chapter explores how framing can either alleviate or intensify stigma—highlighting the importance of strategic communication efforts that focus on structural causes and recovery stories to reduce negative stereotypes, while cautioning against emphasizing personal accountability or risk, which can enforce stigma. The chapter concludes by proposing future research directions to deepen understanding of the framing effect in communication related to the opioid crisis.

4.2 Framing Effects Among the Public

4.2.1 Support for Harm Reduction Interventions

When examining the framing effect on the public, one line of research has focused on public support for harm reduction interventions. This line of research has given considerable attention to the impact of frames on public support for the use of Harm Reduction Centers. These centers provide interventions that have been proven to reduce the spread of communicable diseases (e.g., HIV and Hepatitis C), fatal overdoses, and the number of used and discarded syringes in the community (Barry et al. 2018). Despite the evidence concerning the effectiveness of these interventions, they are still plagued by structural and public stigma toward people with opioid use disorder that stifles support for the interventions among community members. Institutional stigma refers to rules, policies, and practices that limit the opportunities and resources available to people with opioid use disorder (e.g., laws that deprive these people of food, housing assistance or health interventions; Cheetham et al. 2022; Krendl and Perry 2023). Particularly relevant to the operation of Harm Reduction Centers is a federal statute under the Controlled Substances Act that prevents any organization from operating a facility that permits the use of illicit drugs (Boyd and Saleh 2022). This law directly affects the operation of Harm Reduction Centers, which allow individuals to test and use illicit substances while being supervised by trained staff who are readily available to administer overdose prevention medications in the event of an overdose.

Public stigma, on the other hand, is defined as negative views and beliefs that promote prejudice and discrimination against people with opioid use disorder. It spills over into intervention support in ways that complicate the implementation of harm reduction interventions. For instance, when Dupree et al. (2021) interviewed community members about their perceptions and support of opening Harm Reduction Centers in Baltimore, some expressed hesitation to support the measure due to their stigmatizing views about people impacted by drug use disorder. Here, scholars have a unique opportunity to explore how framing techniques may alter community members' perceptions of and support for the use of Harm Reduction Centers.

To answer the question, Barry et al. (2018) conducted a two-condition survey experiment to examine how focusing on safety or prevention when framing Harm Reduction Centers may influence support for their use. During the study, participants in the safety frame condition were shown a message describing these centers using the term "Safe Consumption Sites." Those in the prevention frame condition received the same message except that the label "Overdose Prevention Sites" was used to refer to the centers. The study found that framing these centers as Overdose Prevention Sites versus Safe Consumption Sites was more effective in persuading participants to support their use at the community level. According to the researchers, one reason for the observed framing effect is that the label "Overdose Prevention Sites" emphasizes the reality of death and frames these sites as a clear solution to fatal overdoses. Conversely, referring to these centers as "Safe Consumption Sites" may lead the public to believe that the sites merely aim at making illicit and heavily stigmatized drug use safer for a highly stigmatized group.

While the work of Barry et al. (2018) has been instrumental in bettering our understanding of how the labels assigned to Harm Reduction Centers can influence public support for their use, some researchers have highlighted the need to address nuances in support, as research has shown that support for the use of these facilities can be stifled by Not In My Back Yard (NIMBY) concerns over where these facilities are placed. In other words, some community members may support the use of these facilities at the national level but not in their community (Lofaro and Miller 2021). Building off the work by Barry et al. (2018), Socia et al. (2021) explored whether pairing label frames (i.e., Safe Injection Facilities versus Overdose Prevention Sites) with accompanying information that framed Harm Reduction Centers as either being beneficial for crime control or public health would address differences in support for the use of these facilities at the local and national levels. To answer the question, Socia et al. conducted a national survey experiment with a 2 (facility label: Safe Injection Facility versus Overdose Prevention Site) × 3 (accompanying information: No information, crime control benefits, versus public health benefits) between-subjects design. During the study, two groups of participants were exposed to a message that provided a brief overview of Harm Reduction Centers, using the label of "Safe Injection Facility" or "Overdose Prevention Site." The remaining four groups were given additional information about the centers that emphasized how these facilities could benefit crime control or public health efforts. The study found that when it comes to the framing effect, framing the label mattered more than framing the accompanying information. Specifically, the results showed that, regardless of the information provided, the label "Overdose Prevention Site" was more effective at convincing the public to support the use of Harm Reduction Centers at the local and national levels. However, the label did not overcome NIMBY concerns. Among participants who were exposed to the "Overdose Prevention Site" label, support for the use of these facilities was still higher at the national level than at the local level.

More recently, Johnston and Thompson (2024) explored how compassion, just the fact, safety/security, and harm reduction frames influenced public support for the use of Harm Reduction Centers. Unlike Barry et al. (2018) and Socia et al. (2021), who focused only on framing written text (that is, the labels and information used to describe the facilities), Johnston and Thompson (2024) tested the framing effects of labels, accompanying information, and images. In the study, the compassion frame used the label "Overdose Prevention Program" (OPP). The accompanying information was framed using language that emphasized compassion and empathy for those struggling with opioid use disorder. The two images presented along with the message portrayed individuals in recovery interacting with their loved ones, with the caption that read "OPP extends lives an average of 34 years" or "With OPPs, people are more likely to begin recovery." (Johnston and Thompson 2024, 5). The just the facts frame used the label "Supervised Injection Facilities" to refer to Harm Reduction Centers. The facility description was framed in terms of the effectiveness of the interventions offered (Johnston and Thompson 2024, 6). One of the two images shown in this condition depicted two individuals talking with a caption that read, "Zero fatalities reported." The other was a hemoglobin graphic with the caption, "Stop the spread of HIV" (Johnston and Thompson 2024, 5). Participants in the safety/security frame condition saw the label "Safe Consumption Site" (SCS) and read a facility description that emphasized the importance of community safety. One of the two images included in this condition was that of a young girl walking in a park, with the caption, "Because of SCS, she can walk barefoot in the park." The other image depicted a peaceful neighborhood with the caption, "Because every neighborhood should feel safe" (Johnston and Thompson 2024, 5). Finally, in the harm reduction frame condition, participants were exposed to the label "Harm Reduction Center" (HRC) and a description of the center that highlighted harm reduction principles such as having little to no barrier to treatment access and being welcoming to those impacted by opioid use disorder regardless of where they are in their recovery process. Both images shown in this study condition included healthcare professionals working with patients to provide care with the caption, "HRCs cost 20 times less than a typical rehab program" or "All are welcome night and day" (Johnston and Thompson 2024, 5).

The study found that just the facts and compassion frames were significantly more effective than safety/security and harm reduction frames at increasing public support for the use of Harm Reduction Centers (Johnston and Thompson 2024). The observed persuasive advantage of the compassion frame is consistent with the findings of the studies by Socia et al. (2021) and Barry et al. (2018), which suggest the effectiveness of labeling that emphasizes prevention and the need to save lives. In Johnston and Thompson study (2024), the compassion frame resonated with audience members by speaking to their values concerning the importance of recovery and saving lives. The just the facts frame is effective partly because most people are unaware of how Harm Reduction Centers operate. By educating the public about the efficacy of the interventions provided at these facilities, the frame has the potential to rally public support for the operation of the facilities.

In addition to exploring the framing effect on support for the use of Harm Reduction Centers, researchers have also tested how various message frames may affect public support for the use of Narcan, a lifesaving intervention that has proven to reverse the fatal effects of an opioid overdose. To assess the framing effect on support for this intervention, Bagley et al. (2022) investigated the influence of three framing techniques—that is, gain versus loss frames, labeling individuals with opioid use disorder as "addicts" or "victims," and linguistic assignment of agency—on people's intentions to acquire more information about Narcan, accept a coupon for Narcan, and purchase Narcan. The study found that loss-framed messages were more persuasive than gain-framed messages due to the former's ability to convey greater urgency and severity.

The label attached to individuals with opioid use disorder also shaped behavioral intentions, but in unexpected ways (Bagley et al. 2022). While the "victim" label was expected to elicit more empathy and be more effective, the "addict" label was associated with higher perceptions of Narcan's effectiveness. One possible explanation may be that, unlike the label "victim," which implies fatality and finality, the term "addict" suggests that the individual with opioid use disorder is still alive and potentially responsive to intervention.

Moreover, assignment of linguistic agency was found to play a notable role in shaping threat information processing (Bagley et al. 2022). Messages assigning agency to humans (rather than the opioid threat) heightened perceptions of susceptibility and led to greater intentions to seek information about Narcan. Conversely, assigning agency to the opioid threat elevated perceptions of severity. Overall, the study by Bagley et al. (2022) highlights the nuanced ways in which various message framing techniques—especially gain versus loss frames, labels attached to individuals with opioid use disorder, and linguistic assignment of agency—can shape people's intentions to seek information about and use Narcan.

4.2.2 *Stigma Reduction and Policy Support*

Besides support for harm reduction interventions, another area of inquiry by framing effect scholars is stigma reduction and policy support among the public. After leaving prison, individuals with prior drug convictions, specifically felony drug convictions, often have a hard time reintegrating into communities, having their basic needs (e.g., food and housing) met, and going on to live a healthy and productive life partly due to stigma (Bandara et al. 2020). As Frankel and Depoy remind us, "one of the main barriers to successful acclimation to community following release from incarceration is stigma" (2021, 1). Indeed, Moore et al. (2013) conducted a longitudinal study of 180 incarcerated individuals and discovered evidence that echoed this sentiment. To be more specific, the study found that more than 60% of participants agreed that "people on the outside think once a criminal, always a criminal" and "people on the outside think all criminals are bad people" (Moore et al. 2013, 7).

To improve the well-being of individuals with prior drug convictions, certain policies are implemented at the federal and state levels. For example, the First Step Act (including provisions for sentencing reform and reentry programs) was passed by the Congress in 2018 to reduce the harm caused by the laws that mandate minimum sentencing for drug offenses (Bandara et al. 2020). Furthermore, some states have modified their laws to remove the lifetime ban on food assistance for those with prior drug convictions (Bandara et al. 2020). Nonetheless, stigma still is a key barrier to public support for policies that improve the lives of individuals with prior drug convictions (Bandara et al. 2020). Because of this, scholars have started to explore how framing strategies can be used to influence stigma toward people with prior drug convictions and support for policies that benefit these people.

For example, the study by Bandara et al. (2020) explored how consequence frames may influence stigma and policy support. The study tested the effects of three types of consequence frames (i.e., public safety, impact on children, and social justice) on stigma toward people with prior drug convictions and support for non-punitive legislation. The public safety frame emphasized the potential impact of laws that further criminalize non-violent individuals with a history of drug use on crime/public safety. The impact on children frame highlighted how tough-on-crime laws could affect the well-being of children whose parents are non-violent drug offenders. The social justice frame emphasized the disproportionate negative impact of harsher legislation on marginalized populations and the detrimental influence of post-release challenges on the hardship and disparities these populations face.

The study found that, relative to participants in the control condition, those in the social justice frame condition expressed more support for the elimination of mandatory minimum sentencing for people convicted of felony drug offenses and the removal of the requirements to disclose the criminal history of felony drug offenders on job applications (Bandara et al. 2020). Although the social justice frame increased participants' willingness to live next to someone with a felony drug conviction, it decreased participants' confidence in felony drug offenders' ability to rehabilitate. Like the social justice frame, the impact on children frame also promoted support for the removal of the requirement of reporting felony drug offenses on job applications and increased participants' willingness to live next to someone with a felony drug conviction. Also similar to the social justice frame, the impact on children frame failed to increase participants' confidence in felony drug offenders' capability for rehabilitation. The public safety frame, however, failed to produce any significant changes in stigma or policy support. These findings serve as a reminder that consequence frames can be effective at shifting the public's attributions of responsibility, which is a key factor in reducing stigma (Bandara et al. 2020). For example, the social justice frame highlighted the systemic barriers faced by formerly incarcerated minorities and low-income individuals with prior drug convictions. Similarly, the impact on children frame focused on the impact that reentry struggles can have on children. In both frames, the responsibilities were shifted from individuals who bear the stigma to external factors such as systemic barriers, which helped reduce stigma. Finally, the impact on children frame brought people's attention to the reality that punitive policies harm not only formerly incarcerated individuals but also their children. Thus, this type of frame can be instrumental in humanizing a stigmatized population.

Up until recently, research into the framing effect on stigma has largely focused on depictions of the opioid crisis more broadly. Scant attention has been paid to the impact of media framing of the opioid crisis in rural areas on stigma toward individuals with opioid use disorder. Media framing of the rural opioid crisis has mainly emphasized the growth or spread of the opioid epidemic and the need for more resources in these areas (Lawson et al. 2021). Rural communities face unique access barriers that largely stem from systemic poverty and/or the geographical layout of these communities (Lawson et al. 2021). For example, a lack of public transportation combined with the long distances travel required for most people to seek care and treatment for opioid use disorder creates a daunting access barrier in rural communities (Stopka et al. 2024). Thus, it's important for scholars to explore how framing of the rural opioid crisis can influence stigma toward individuals with opioid use disorder among the public.

To answer the question, Lawson et al. (2021) tested the effects of three types of frames—that is, individual depiction, causal, and consequences frames. The individual depiction frame included individuals' stories of addiction and recovery in rural America. The causal frame emphasized the causal contributions of the pharmaceutical industry and prescribers of opioid drugs to the rural opioid crisis. The consequence frame highlighted the financial burden that rural communities are shouldering due to the opioid crisis. The researchers found that, relative to the causal and consequence frames, the individual depiction frame was effective at reducing stigma toward individuals with opioid use disorder (Lawson et al. 2021). A primary reason for the effectiveness of the individual depiction frame is linked to the inclusion of information about recovery. In fact, research has shown that positive information such as that provided by stories or messages about recovery is effective at reducing stigma toward individuals with opioid use disorder (Livingston et al. 2012).

In summary, a growing body of research has highlighted the crucial role that framing can play in shaping public support for harm reduction interventions, stigma toward individuals with opioid use disorder, and attitudes toward policies that benefit these individuals. While understanding the framing effect among the public is valuable, it is also important to explore how framing issues related to the opioid crisis may influence the perceptions, attitudes, and behaviors of specific populations. Thus, the next three sections will examine the framing effects on policymakers, law enforcements, and White Americans.

4.3 Framing Effects Among Policymakers

One population that is understudied by framing effect research is policymakers. This is ironic given that framing is a core component of theories in policymaking. For example, Punctuated Equilibrium Theory posits that major policy shifts occur in part due to how social problems are framed or reframed in society (Jones and Baumgartner 2004). To be clear, some scholars have outlined several reasons as to why message framing may not have intended effects among policymakers (Bergan et al. 2023). Specifically, they contend that, relative to the general public, policymakers tend to hold stronger attitudes toward social issues, and the framing effect is less likely to occur among individuals with strong attitudes. Moreover, lawmakers' policy attitudes are heavily influenced by their political party because they are incentivized to take stands that align with their party's agenda, which makes them less susceptible to the influence of framing. However, there is evidence suggesting that policymakers may be subjective to the influence of framing due to their high level of political knowledge. For example, Druckman and Nelson (2003) showed that when controlling for prior attitudes, framing effects were more evident among participants with more political knowledge.

Moreover, framing issues related to the opioid crisis in ways that are consistent with how the general public perceives them may be of relevance to policymakers (Bergan et al. 2023). Here, macro-frames can play a pivotal role. Macro-frames are messages that reflect how the general public defines an issue, what components of that issue are more pronounced to the public, and how the public attributes responsibility related to the issue. Given that macro-frames reflect the public's perception, policymakers may have an incentive to make sure that their policy decisions align with the macro-framing of important social and public health issues. To explore the impacts of macro-frames on causal attributions and policy support related to the opioid crisis among lawmakers, Bergan et al. (2023) conducted an experiment among policymakers in Illinois, a state heavily impacted by the crisis. The study had a 3 (framing messages: societal, individual, or control) by 3 (macro-level frames: societal responsibility, individual responsibility, or control) between-subjects design. The first set of frames either highlighted the societal responsibility for the opioid crisis (i.e., societal frame) or portrayed an individual affected by the crisis (i.e., individual frame). The second set of frames, macro-frames, emphasized the public belief in either societal (i.e., societal macro-frame) or individuals' (e.g., doctors or patients) responsibility (i.e., individual macro-frame) for combating the opioid crisis.

While none of the frames had a significant effect on policy support among lawmakers, the societal frame did impact policymakers' attributions of responsibility for the opioid crisis and their perceptions of responsibility attributions by the public (Bergan et al. 2023). Specifically, the study found that when policymakers were exposed to the societal frame, they were more likely to attribute the cause of the opioid crisis to societal factors and perceive the public to attribute more responsibility to society. These findings are consistent with prior research showing that message frames that focus on the larger societal context are effective at persuading individuals that the causes of a social issue are rooted in society (Iyengar 1996).

4.4 Framing Effects Among Law Enforcement

Another population that is understudied by framing effect research related to the opioid crisis is law enforcement officials. When it comes to implementing evidence-based interventions such as syringe exchange programs or medication-assisted treatments, law enforcement officers can hinder these efforts (Raychaudhuri et al. 2023). For example, research shows that most police responses to opioid overdoses lead to arrest rather than treatment. Moreover, drug seizures carried out by law enforcement officers have proven to increase the number of fatal overdoses (Raychaudhuri et al. 2023). A primary driver of these negative interactions between law enforcement officers and individuals with drug use disorder is stigma toward the latter. In fact, research shows that younger police officers, those with lower levels of educational attainment, and those who hold beliefs that addiction is a moral failing are more likely to subject people with drug use disorder to stigmatization than to refer them to treatment (Del Pozo et al. 2024a).

Moreover, tension exists between law enforcement's mission of protecting public safety (e.g., saving lives) and their legal duty (Lloyd et al. 2023). On one hand, research shows that police officers strongly feel that they can play a positive role in preventing drug overdose deaths, which is consistent with their public safety mission (Del Pozo et al. 2024a). On the other hand, their legal duties require them to execute arrest warrants, seize illicit drugs, and maintain social order. Thus, it is important for law enforcement officers to reconcile their public safety mission and legal duties in response to drug-related incidents.

While law enforcement officers have great discretion in their responses to drug-related incidents (Del Pozo et al. 2024b), leaders in law enforcement organizations (e.g., police chiefs) have the power to influence police officers' behaviors in ways that facilitate harm reduction efforts (Marotta et al. 2023). For this reason, Del Pozo et al. (2024a) conducted an experiment to explore how framing techniques may influence police chiefs' perceptions of the mission of police officers, trust in officers in recovery from opioid use disorder, and support for harm reduction interventions. During the study, police chiefs answered one of the two versions of a questionnaire with 37 questions, 9 of which adopted either a health (using words and phrases such as "Overdose Prevention Sites," "public health," and "reduce harm") or safety frame ("Safe Injection Sites," "public safety," and "reduce overdose death and injury").

The findings of the study suggest that framing matters when engaging police officials (Del Pozo et al. 2024a). Although police chiefs were significantly more likely to support the use of Harm Reduction Centers when they were framed as "Overdose Prevention Sites" (health frame) as opposed to "Safe Injection Sites" (safety frame), the differences in police chiefs' responses to the two versions of the questionnaire demonstrated their preference for interventions being framed as benefiting public safety as opposed to public health. For example, police chiefs were significantly more likely to agree that their mission was to protect public safety than to protect public health. They were more inclined to support police officers distributing Narcan on patrol if the measure was "shown to reduce overdose death and injury" (safety frame) than if it was shown to "reduce harm" (health frame). Moreover, the chiefs showed greater support for the Good Samaritan laws (that protect people from arrest when they call 911 to report a drug overdose) when the law was described using the safety frame (i.e., they "save lives") instead of the health frame (i.e., they "reduce harm").

Finally, police chiefs expressed significantly more trust in police officers in recovery from opioid use disorder when the safety, as opposed to health, frame was used partly because the health frame mentioned that the recovery involved the medication buprenorphine while the safety frame did not (Del Pozo et al. 2024a). This framing effect can be explained by what Madden (2019) has coined as "intervention stigma." Unlike traditional forms of stigma that place a mark upon an individual because of their health status or physical characteristics, intervention stigma leads to the stigmatization of patients and providers of controversial interventions (Madden 2019). Research has shown that, despite the evidence showing that medication-assisted treatment is effective at helping individuals with opioid use disorder recover, stigma still exists for the treatment in communities where people believe that medication-assisted treatment simply allows patients to swap out one drug for another (Madden 2019). This stigmatizing perception leads to a lack of respect for this type of recovery treatment. The observed negative impact of the health frame (which mentioned medication-assisted recovery) on trust in police officers in recovery from opioid use disorder (Del Pozo et al. 2024a) indicates that the frame may have activated intervention stigma toward users of medication-assisted treatment, which in turn lowered police chiefs' trust in officers in recovery from opioid use disorder.

Taken together, the study by Del Pozo et al. (2024a) not only extends the findings from earlier studies (Barry et al. 2018; Socia et al. 2021) into a different population but also provides new insights into the framing effect among law enforcement. Given the work of Barry et al. (2018) and Socia et al. (2021), it is not surprising that support for Harm Reduction Centers was higher among police chiefs who were exposed to the frame that labeled the facilities as Overdose Prevention Sites than among those exposed to the frame that referred to the facilities as Safe Injection Sites. Nonetheless, the finding extends the work of Barry et al. (2018) and Socia et al. (2021) by showing that framing that emphasizes prevention can also be effective among police officials when attempting to persuade them to support the operation of Harm Reduction Centers (Del Pozo et al. 2024a). More importantly, the study by Del Pozo et al. (2024a) suggests that framing that emphasizes safety as opposed to health resonates more with police officials and may be more effective at mobilizing their support for harm reduction interventions (e.g., distributing Narcan).

4.5 Framing Effects Among White Americans

4.5.1 Loser Perceptions and Policy Support

While opioid use disorder is widely understood to be a public health issue that can impact anyone regardless of their racial/ethnic identity, the media often frame this issue as one that primarily impacts White Americans (Netherland and Hansen 2016) because there is data to suggest that the opioid crisis is claiming more lives among Whites than among other racial groups (Gollust and Miller 2020). For example, in 2017 37,113 White Americans died from an opioid overdose. That same year, only 5513 Black Americans died of an opioid overdose.

While comparative frames—those emphasizing a higher prevalence of opioid dependence and overdose among Whites than among other racial/ethnic groups—have played a hand in whitewashing the opioid crisis, these types of frames have also been used to explain why the opioid crisis is framed as an "epidemic" (that is, a public health issue). For example, in a 2018 article from *the New York Times*, a writer uses a comparative frame to highlight the higher incidence of neonatal abstinence syndrome among White newborns whose mothers have a history of opioid dependence. The writer then goes on to state, "Indeed, the perception of our opioid crisis as an epidemic, rather than a racial pathology, owes much to the fact that White Americans have been hard hit" (Gollust and Miller 2020, 247). For this reason, there is increased interest in understanding how framing the opioid crisis may affect White individuals' perceptions that they are on the losing side of public health policy related to the crisis (Gollust and Miller 2020). Understanding the framing effect on loser perceptions is important because a growing body of research shows that perceiving oneself as a political loser can influence political attitudes and behaviors. For example, in her book *White Identity Politics*, Ashley Jardina opines that loser perceptions among Whites are strong predictors of their willingness to support policies and political actors that can make "Make America Great Again" (cited in Gollust and Miller 2020, 243).

Within the context of the opioid crisis, the work of Gollust and Miller (2020) provides insights into how various framing techniques may shape White Americans' loser perceptions and policy support. In their study, White participants were randomly assigned to one of three study conditions—the control, absolute frame, and comparative frame conditions. Participants in the control condition received no message. Those in the absolute frame condition read an article that reported the high opioid overdose mortality rates among Whites. Participants in the comparative frame condition saw an article suggesting that the opioid crisis poses a greater threat to White Americans than to Black Americans by showing the differences in opioid overdose mortality rates across the two racial groups. The study found that, relative to White participants in the control condition, those in the comparative frame condition were more likely to feel that the White race was on the losing side of public health policy. Participants in the absolute frame condition, on the other hand, were more likely than those in the control condition to support public health-oriented policy measures to tackle the opioid crisis (that is, more empathetic policy). Collectively, these findings indicate that media framing of the impact of the opioid crisis on White Americans can have important implications for Whites' perceptions of themselves and policy support.

4.5.2 Treatment Support

Building off the work by Gollust and Miller (2020), Raychaudhuri et al. (2023) explored the impacts of different framing techniques (that is, valence and race frames) on White Americans' support for government-funded treatment programs (over punishment) that benefit people with opioid use disorder. In the study, valence frames are defined as, "a set of positive or negative framing elements consisting of external or individual blame, deserving or underserving users, and a focus on the target's suffering versus their crime" (Raychaudhuri et al. 2023, 169). Race frames were operationalized by images of a Black or White individual presented along with a sympathetic portrayal of a person with opioid use disorder (i.e., the positive valence frame) or an unsympathetic portrayal (i.e., the negative valence frame).

The study found that a sympathetic portrayal (i.e., the positive frame) of a person with opioid use disorder, regardless of the person's race, increased White participants' support for treatment programs (Raychaudhuri et al. 2023). Moreover, the observed positive impact of the sympathetic portrayal was larger in size when the person being portrayed was White, due to study participants' racially selective sympathy rooted in their racial identity. The findings have important policy implications. Specifically, they suggest that framing the opioid crisis as a public health crisis that victimizes White Americans (as opposed to racial minorities) may better rally public support for government-funded treatment programs and, therefore, allow policymakers to focus more on public health-oriented rather than punitive solutions to the crisis (Raychaudhuri et al. 2023).

4.6 Directions for Future Research

The framing effect research reviewed in this chapter suggests some promising avenues for future research. One important area for future research involves a comprehensive exploration of the framing effect among distinct ethnic/racial groups. Although several studies have explored the effects of various frames (i.e., absolute, comparative, race, and valence frames) on White participants' willingness to support public health-oriented policy/ interventions related to the opioid crisis (Gollust and Miller 2020; Raychaudhuri et al. 2023), no studies have examined the effects of these or other frames on Black or Non-White Hispanic Americans. This gap in the literature needs to be addressed because, while rates of drug overdose have declined overall in the past couple of years, they have increased for Black and Hispanic Americans (Garnett and Miniño 2024; Henderson 2024). Along the same lines, framing effect studies should also explore how various framing techniques may influence Native Hawaiians or other Pacific Islanders because this group experienced the largest increase in rates of overdose from 2022 to 2023 (Garnett and Miniño 2024).

Beyond the framing effect on racial minorities, future research may also explore whether frames other than those tested by previous studies (e.g., health versus safety frames, Del Pozo et al. 2024b; individual versus societal frames, Bergan et al. 2023) may be effective in shaping the beliefs, attitudes, opinions, and behavior of policymakers or law enforcement. For example, such research could explore the extent to which causal frames and/or positive versus negative frames may shape police officers' causal perceptions of opioid use disorder. It is also important to investigate how framing the opioid crisis and people with opioid use disorder may reduce stigma among policymakers and police officers, as their stigmatizing views could undermine their support for harm reduction interventions (Kennedy-Hendricks et al. 2017). The stigmatizing view of police officers could also negatively affect their interaction with individuals suffering from opioid use disorder, leading to more punitive (e.g., arrest) than empathetic responses (e.g., treatment referrals) to opioid overdose incidents and causing more harm to those with opioid use disorder. Hence, understanding how to leverage various framing techniques to combat stigma among lawmakers and police officers is crucial for the success of harm reduction efforts.

Despite evidence showing that syringe exchange programs can play a crucial role in reducing instances of overdose and the spread of communicable diseases such as HIV and Hepatitis C, 11 states in the United States currently outlaw such programs (KFF, 2025). With the only exception of the study by Del Pozo et al. (2024b), which examined the influence of health versus safety frames on police officials' support for the intervention, little research has been done to explore how framing techniques may contribute to the acceptance of empirically supported interventions and promote the legalization of such interventions. Thus, future studies could explore how frames that highlight evidence showing the effectiveness of harm reduction interventions (e.g., syringe exchange programs) at the individual and community level may influence support for the interventions among policymakers, law enforcement, and the public.

Moreover, researchers could examine whether fiscally conservative frames (i.e., those that emphasize the financial savings/benefits of an intervention) are more effective than frames that highlight an individual's recovery journey in persuading lawmakers to support legislation that minimizes the harm caused by the opioid crisis. Researchers may also identify and test the influence of frames aligned with policymakers' motivations (e.g., electoral incentives, ideological commitments, and constituent demands) on their policy decisions. Comparative studies that examine the impacts of various frames among lawmakers across levels of government and affiliated with different political parties could further clarify effective framing approaches for different audiences.

Future framing effect studies should also explore understudied outcome variables such as NIMBY (Not In My Backyard) sentiment and backing politicians promoting specific policies. Such research could also investigate the framing effect on support for medication-assisted treatment. As an evidence-based solution, medication-assisted treatment programs prescribe one of two substances, methadone or buprenorphine, to treat individuals with opioid use disorder. The treatments have been proven to reduce the risk of overdose, improve treatment retention, and lower drug-related crimes in communities (Madden 2019). Despite their effectiveness, intervention stigma plagues the treatments in ways that limit their use. For this reason, future framing effect studies should explore the types of frames that can be used to reduce stigma toward medication-assisted treatments and other interventions whose usage is limited by intervention stigma (e.g., syringe exchange programs and overdose prevention sites).

In addition to intervention stigma, researchers should also explore the framing effect on other types of understudied stigma such as internalized (or self) stigma and structural (or institutional) stigma (Cheetham et al. 2022; Krendl and Perry 2023). Internalized stigma related to opioid use disorder are negative thoughts and feelings (e.g., shame) about oneself due to one's identity as a person with opioid use disorder. Framing effect research could explore how using different ways to frame recovery may influence internalized stigma among individuals with opioid use disorder. Such research could also examine whether the frames under study may produce different effects across various populations (e.g., White versus Black individuals with opioid use disorder). Beyond this, researchers could assess whether and how positive/negative frames or race frames of the opioid crisis may influence support for structural stigma among the public and policymakers. By doing so, they would answer the call to conduct more research on structural stigma (Hatzenbuehler 2016).

Thus far, most framing effect research in the context of the opioid crisis has focused exclusively on immediate or short-term effects (Bandara et al. 2020; Gollust and Miller 2020; Del Pozo et al. 2024b; Johnston and Thompson 2024), which raises the question of how the effect may change over time. Given that promoting enduring attitudinal and behavioral changes is often the goal of health communication, it is important for researchers to conduct longitudinal studies to track framing effects on message receivers' beliefs, attitudes, policy preferences, and behaviors over an extended period of time. Such studies could also identify factors that contribute to the persistence of framing effects (e.g., repeated exposure, integration of the framing into pre-existing belief systems, and social reinforcement) or their attenuation (e.g., personal experiences and cognitive dissonance).

Given that the modern media environment allows individuals to acquire information from multiple sources that often frame the same issue/topic differently, it is important for future research to explore how multiple competing frames interact to influence the audience. Investigating how individuals cognitively manage these competing frames—whether they selectively attend to congruent information, reconcile opposing perspectives, or experience cognitive overload—could provide a deeper understanding of the framing effect. For example, researchers could explore the effects of different emphasis frames that portray recovery as abstinence-only versus being inclusive of medication-assisted treatment on attitudes toward the treatment and people in recovery. These researchers could also investigate the influence of competing frames that emphasize racial equality versus colorblind approaches to treating opioid use disorder among audiences with various racial/ethical identities. Furthermore, investigating the efficacy of counter-framing strategies to mitigate the influence of dominant, potentially harmful frames, about the opioid crisis and individuals with opioid use disorder could enhance our understanding of effective counter-messaging tactics.

The growth in popularity of digital and social media platforms represents another fertile area for future framing research. Traditional framing effect research is conducted primarily in broadcast and print media contexts, often neglecting the nuances introduced by digital and social media platforms. These platforms differ significantly from traditional media as they allow for the rapid dissemination of messages with various frames and hashtags, enable user-generated content, and create algorithmically driven echo chambers. For this reason, researchers could investigate the framing effect of viral hashtags like #opioidcrisis on public perceptions of the issue, or how algorithmic amplification of certain narratives and/or user comments could shape how the issues and people related to the opioid crisis are framed in the discourses on digital and social media platforms. Moreover, studying the number of likes and shares that messages adopting various frames receive may reveal the types of frames that resonate with the public and could potentially have greater impacts on message receivers' perceptions, beliefs, attitudes, and behavior. This line of inquiry might also explore specific features of frames that enhance their virality or how echo chambers reinforce the influence of existing frames, thereby leading to polarized perceptions of topics such as opioid use disorder or public health-oriented interventions.

Historically, framing effect research has predominantly centered on textual content, despite the powerful influence that visual imagery and nonverbal elements exert on perceptions and emotions (Guenther et al., 2021). Thus, exploring the framing effect of visual and nonverbal elements should be one of the areas of future research. Such research should systematically investigate how visual frames, such as images depicting affected individuals or highlighting systemic contexts, influence audiences independently and in conjunction with textual content. Studying the interplay between visual and textual framing could offer particularly potent insights, illuminating the conditions under which visual framing reinforces, contradicts, or moderates the framing effect of text. Moreover, the cognitive and emotional processing mechanisms triggered by visual stimuli warrant further examination, particularly in terms of their implications for memory retention and behavioral intentions. Future research on visual and nonverbal framing should also evaluate its impacts among and across various populations. For instance, investigating whether certain visual or nonverbal frames are more effective with White versus non-White populations or police chiefs versus lower-ranked police officers.

As research into the framing effect continues to evolve, scholars increasingly recognize the importance of addressing the ethical considerations that come with using various framing techniques (Bagley et al. 2022). When framing is employed deliberately for strategic purposes, such as shaping public attitudes toward complex and sensitive issues (e.g., stigma and substance use disorder), ethical concerns become particularly salient. For this reason, practitioners must scrutinize their practices, ensuring that their use of framing aligns with ethical principles and social responsibilities. To explore best practices, researchers should explicitly investigate and delineate the ethical boundaries and responsibilities associated with strategic framing. This could include promoting transparency in the framing process, actively avoiding manipulative tactics or the dissemination of misinformation, and striving to strike a balance between the pursuit of message effectiveness and the maintenance of ethical integrity. Researchers could also evaluate the ethical implications of various framing techniques by soliciting insights from a diverse array of stakeholders—including members of the general public, individuals with opioid use disorder, advocacy groups, policymakers, and ethicists. Finally, future studies should examine potential unintended consequences of the deployment of various framing techniques, such as reinforcing stereotypes, fostering polarization, or eroding public trust. By taking into account ethical considerations associated with strategic framing uncovered by framing effect research, practitioners could ensure that their efforts would contribute positively to societal well-being and uphold democratic values.

By expanding framing effect research in the directions listed here, future studies will significantly improve our understanding of the framing effect in the context of the opioid crisis. These endeavors will make valuable contributions to the development of effective, ethical, and nuanced communication strategies that address the complex societal challenges posed by the crisis, inform public policy debates, and foster greater public awareness and acceptance of critical health and social interventions aimed at combating the crisis.

References

Bagley, Braden Hale, Kathryn Anthony, and Steven Venette. 2022. Framing, Agency, and Optimistic Bias: Message Design Considerations for the Opioid Crisis. *Communication Research and Practice* 8 (4): 347–363. https://doi.org/10.1080/22041451.2022.2143665.

Bandara, Sachini N., Emma E. McGinty, and Colleen L. Barry. 2020. Message Framing to Reduce Stigma and Increase Support for Policies to Improve the Wellbeing of People with Prior Drug Convictions. *International Journal of Drug Policy* 76:102643. https://doi.org/10.1016/j.drugpo.2019.102643.

Barry, Colleen L., Susan G. Sherman, and Emma E. McGinty. 2018. Language Matters in Combatting the Opioid Epidemic: Safe Consumption Sites versus Overdose Prevention Sites. *American Journal of Public Health* 108 (9): 1157–1159. https://doi.org/10.2105/AJPH.2018.304588.

Bergan, Daniel E., Alan Rojas, Ian Briggs, and Emily Andersen. 2023. Framing and Policymaker Evaluations of the Opioid Crisis. *Health Communication* 38 (12): 2604–2616. https://doi.org/10.1080/10410236.2022.2093555.

Boyd, Chelsea, and Mazen Saleh. (2022). Overdose Prevention Centers and the Federal 'Crack House Statute.' *R Street Institute* (blog), February 16. https://www.rstreet.org/research/overdose-prevention-centers-and-the-federal-crack-house-statute/.

Cheetham, Ali, Louisa Picco, Anthony Barnett, Dan I. Lubman, and Suzanne Nielsen. 2022. The Impact of Stigma on People with Opioid Use Disorder, Opioid Treatment, and Policy. *Substance Abuse and Rehabilitation* 13:1–12. https://doi.org/10.2147/SAR.S304566.

Collins, Alexandra B., Jade Boyd, Hannah L. F. Cooper, and Ryan McNeil. 2019. The Intersectional Risk Environment of People Who Use Drugs. *Social Science & Medicine* 234:112384. https://doi.org/10.1016/j.socscimed.2019.112384.

Del Pozo, Brandon, Jessica Reichert, Kaitlin Martins, and Bruce Taylor. 2024a. Police Use of Discretion in Encounters with People with Opioid Use Disorder: A Study of Illinois Police Officers. *Journal of Police and Criminal Psychology* 39, no. 1:141–156. https://doi.org/10.1007/s11896-023-09628-9.

Del Pozo, Brandon, Saba Rouhani, M. H. Amelia Bailey, Kaitlin F. Clark, Fatema Z. Martins, Danielle Atkins Ahmed, and Barbara Andraka-Christou. 2024b. The Effects of Message Framing on US Police Chiefs' Support for Interventions for Opioid Use Disorder: A Randomized Survey Experiment. *Health & Justice* 12 (1): 50. https://doi.org/10.1186/s40352-024-00306-4.

Druckman, James N., and Kjersten R. Nelson. 2003. Framing and Deliberation: How Citizens' Conversations Limit Elite Influence. *American Journal of Political Science* 47 (4): 729–745. https://doi.org/10.1111/1540-5907.00051.

Dupree, Timothy, Caroline Wood, Brace Andrea. (2021) Understanding the Stigma and Feasibility of Opening a Safe Injection Facility in Baltimore City: A Qualitative Case Study The Qualitative Report. https://doi.org/10.46743/2160-3715/2021.4689

Frankel, Amy, and Elizabeth DePoy. (2021). Thoughts Beyond Stigma-Implications for Change Reflected in the Voices of Previously Incarcerated Citizens, November 14. https://doi.org/10.21428/cb6ab371.a29241e4

Garnett, Matthew, and Arialdi Miniño. (2024). Drug Overdose Deaths in the United States, 2003–2023. *Centers for Disease Control and Prevention*, December 19. https://www.cdc.gov/nchs/products/databriefs/db522.htm

Gollust, Sarah E., and Joanne M. Miller. 2020. Framing the Opioid Crisis: Do Racial Frames Shape Beliefs of Whites Losing Ground? *Journal of Health Politics, Policy and Law* 45 (2): 241–276. https://doi.org/10.1215/03616878-8004874.

Guenther, Lars, Maria Gaertner, and Jessica Zeitz. 2021. Framing as a Concept for Health Communication: A Systematic Review. *Health Communication* 36 (7): 891–899. https://doi.org/10.1080/10410236.2020.1723048.

Hatzenbuehler, Mark L. 2016. Structural Stigma and Health Inequalities: Research Evidence and Implications for Psychological Science. *The American Psychologist* 71 (8): 742–751. https://doi.org/10.1037/amp0000068.

Henderson, Tim. (2024). Overdose Deaths Are Rising among Black and Indigenous Americans Stateline. *Stateline* (blog), October 29. https://stateline.org/2024/10/29/overdose-deaths-are-rising-among-black-and-indigenous-americans/.

Iyengar, Shanto. 1996. Framing Responsibility for Political Issues. *The ANNALS of the American Academy of Political and Social Science* 546 (1): 59–70. https://doi.org/10.1177/0002716296546001006.

Johnston, Jennifer B., and Kaya A. Thompson. 2024. The Name and Frame Matters When It Comes to Public Support of Opioid Prevention Programs. *International Journal of Drug Policy* 123:104282. https://doi.org/10.1016/j.drugpo.2023.104282.

Jones, B. D. (2004) A Model of Choice for Public Policy Journal of Public Administration Research and Theory 15(3) 325-351. https://doi.org/10.1093/jopart/mui018

Kennedy-Hendricks, Alene, Colleen L. Barry, Sarah E. Gollust, Margaret E. Ensminger, Margaret S. Chisolm, and Emma E. McGinty. 2017. Social Stigma toward Persons with Prescription Opioid Use Disorder: Associations with Public Support for Punitive and Public Health-Oriented Policies. *Psychiatric Services* 68 (5): 462–469. https://doi.org/10.1176/appi.ps.201600056.

KFF. (2025). Sterile Syringe Exchange Programs. https://www.kff.org/hivaids/state-indicator/syringe-exchange-programs/.

Krendl, Anne C., and Brea L. Perry. 2023. Stigma toward Substance Dependence: Causes, Consequences, and Potential Interventions. *Psychological Science in the Public Interest* 24 (2): 90–126. https://doi.org/10.1177/15291006231198193.

Lawson, Cara, Courtney Meyers, Amber McCord, Erica Irlbeck, and Amy Boren. 2021. Individual Depictions, Causes, and Consequences: Effects of Media Frames on Perceptions toward the Rural Opioid Epidemic. *Journal of Applied Communications* 105 (2): 4. https://doi.org/10.4148/1051-0834.2377.

Livingston, James D., Teresa Milne, Mei Lan Fang, and Erica Amari. 2012. The Effectiveness of Interventions for Reducing Stigma Related to Substance Use Disorders: A Systematic Review. *Addiction* 107 (1): 39–50. https://doi.org/10.1111/j.1360-0443.2011.03601.x.

Lloyd, Danielle, Kirsten Rowe, Shu-Yin John Leung, Elham Pourtaher, and Kitty Gelberg. 2023. 'It's Just Another Tool on My Toolbelt': New York State Law Enforcement Officer Experiences Administering Naloxone. *Harm Reduction Journal* 20 (1): 29. https://doi.org/10.1186/s12954-023-00748-3.

Lofaro, Ryan J., and Miller, Hugh T. (2021) Narrative Politics in Policy Discourse: The Debate Over Safe Injection Sites in Philadelphia Pennsylvania Contemporary Drug Problems 48(1) 75-95. https://doi.org/10.1177/0091450921993821

Madden, Erin Fanning. 2019. Intervention Stigma: How Medication-Assisted Treatment Marginalizes Patients and Providers. *Social Science & Medicine* 232:324–331. https://doi.org/10.1016/j.socscimed.2019.05.027.

Marotta Phillip L., del Pozo, B., Baker P, et al. (2023) Unlocking deflection: The role of supervisor support in police officer willingness to refer people who inject drugs to harm reduction services International Journal of Drug Policy 121104188. https://doi.org/10.1016/j.drugpo.2023.104188

Moore, Kelly, Jeffrey Stuewig, and June Tangney. 2013. Jail Inmates' Perceived and Anticipated Stigma: Implications for Post-Release Functioning. *Self and Identity* 12 (5): 527–547. https://doi.org/10.1080/15298868.2012.702425.

Netherland, J., and Hansen, Helena B. (2016) The War on Drugs That Wasn't: Wasted Whiteness "Dirty Doctors" and Race in Media Coverage of Prescription Opioid Misuse Culture Medicine and Psychiatry 40(4) 664–686. https://doi.org/10.1007/s11013-016-9496-5

Raychaudhuri, Tanika, Tali Mendelberg, and Anne McDonough. 2023. The Political Effects of Opioid Addiction Frames. *The Journal of Politics* 85 (1): 166–177. https://doi.org/10.1086/720326.

Socia, Kelly M., Rebecca Stone, Wilson R. Palacios, and John Cluverius. 2021. Focus on Prevention: The Public Is More Supportive of 'Overdose Prevention Sites' than They Are of 'Safe Injection Facilities'. *Criminology & Public Policy* 20 (4): 729–754. https://doi.org/10.1111/1745-9133.12566.

Spencer, M. R., Garnett, M. F., & Minino, A. M. (2023, December 21). Drug Overdose Deaths in the United States, 2002–2022.

Stopka, Thomas J., A. T. Estadt, G. Leichtling, et al. 2024. Barriers to Opioid Use Disorder Treatment among People Who Use Drugs in the Rural United States: A Qualitative, Multi-Site Study. *Social Science & Medicine* 346:116660. https://doi.org/10.1016/j.socscimed.2024.116660.

CHAPTER 5

U.S. Newspaper Frames of Chronic Pain in Coverage of the Opioid Crisis, 2012–2022

Elizabeth A. Hintz, Lili R. Romann, and Jacqueline N. Gunning

5.1 Introduction

This chapter reviews how U.S. newspapers framed *chronic pain* (pain persisting ≥ 6 months) in coverage of the opioid crisis between 2012 and 2022 (International Association for the Study of Pain 2024). Chronic pain afflicts one in five U.S. adults and is the leading cause of disability globally (Theo Vos et al. 2016, 1545–1602; Zelaya et al. 2020, 1–8). In the U.S., an epidemic of un(der)treated chronic pain emerged in response to the curtailing of opioid prescribing (Matthias et al. 2020, 1239–1247). Chronic pain and the opioid epidemic are closely linked, and the simultaneous crises of opioids and un(der)treated chronic pain have been referred

E. A. Hintz (✉) • L. R. Romann
Department of Communication, University of Connecticut, Storrs, CT, USA
e-mail: Elizabeth.hintz@uconn.edu; lili.romann@uconn.edu

J. N. Gunning
School of Communication and Journalism, Auburn University, Auburn, AL, USA
e-mail: jacqueline.gunning@uconn.edu

X. Cao (ed.), *Fighting the Opioid Crisis with Communication*,
https://doi.org/10.1007/978-3-032-31162-7_5

to as a "syndemic" (i.e., spiraling dual epidemics; Gunning et al. 2024, 1–12). As Marsha Stanton of *The Deseret News* (Utah) wrote, "The nation is in the middle of an opioid abuse crisis. But we are also in the throes of a chronic pain crisis. The causes of both crises are intertwined, and one can't be addressed while the other is ignored" (Stanton 2017). Despite this, and although ample research has examined news coverage of the opioid epidemic itself, depictions of chronic pain and chronic pain patients—who are marginalized in conversations about the opioid crisis and directly affected by shifting opioid prescribing policies crafted to mitigate that crisis—within such coverage remain underexplored.

Addressing this gap, the current chapter reports on the findings of a comprehensive content analysis of a decade of U.S. newspaper articles ($N = 492$) on the opioid epidemic which also discussed chronic pain (published between 2012 and 2022). Guided by framing theory, this chapter explores how U.S. newspapers selected and presented (framed) particular and salient aspects of chronic pain in coverage of the opioid crisis (Entman 1993, 51–58). Employing media frame analysis, our goal was to identify the (a) dominant frames employed to characterize chronic pain (patients), (b) major "characters" represented (individual people, organizations, and other entities), as well as (c) significant events reported within such news coverage (Giles and Shaw 2009, 375–393). This chapter uses exemplars from news articles included in the final sample to illustrate our findings.

5.2 Content Analysis Procedures

To arrive at our final sample ($N = 492$), we searched NexisUni for English-language, U.S. newspaper articles categorized as "News." We then used a Boolean operator to search specifically for articles mentioning both "chronic pain" and at least one synonym for the opioid crisis utilized in materials published by the Centers for Disease Control and Prevention (CDC 2025; i.e., at least one of the following: "opioid crisis," "opioid epidemic," or "opioid overdose epidemic"), leaving us with an initial sample of 573 articles. We removed 81 duplicate articles (i.e., newswire publications appearing in multiple outlets but not differing by more than 50 words[5]) and inaccessible external links, leaving us with a final sample of 492 articles. Articles ranged in length from 108 to 4922 ($M = 964$; $SD = 632$) words.

After finalizing the sample, we developed and refined the codebook following a process of inductive thematic analysis, guided by the concepts from media frame analysis (i.e., dominant frames, characters, and significant events), as well as the dominant frame types identified by Entman (1993, 51–58). A full description of the content analytic procedures we followed can be found in Gunning et al. 2024 (3122–3133).

We then followed the established content analytic guidelines to train coders (i.e., the second and third authors) and establish inter-rater reliability (Neuendorff 2011; Krippendorff 2018) using Krippendorff's alpha (KALPHA; Hayes and Krippendorff 2007). The two coders were trained over a period of six months using 20% of the total dataset to achieve high reliability (KALPHA > 0.80) on all dominant frames, characters, and significant event types. Where articles included multiple potential dominant frame types (e.g., a newspaper article utilizing the consequence frame also featuring a human-interest story), each article was assigned to a singular dominant frame category via an iterative and deliberative process among the coders. The coders frequently met to discuss disagreements during the training period and resolved each dispute with modifications to the codebook to avoid recurrence of the same dispute. After reliability was achieved on each code in the codebook, the remainder of the sample was divided equally for independent coding by the two coders.

5.3 Dominant Frames of Chronic Pain (Patients) in Newspaper Opioid Crisis Coverage

Our analysis identified four dominant frames used to characterize chronic pain (patients) within U.S. newspaper coverage of the opioid crisis between 2012 and 2022.

5.3.1 The Consequence Frame

The *consequence* frame (n = 146, 29.7%) appeared when newspapers broadly emphasized the effects of the opioid epidemic on chronic pain patients. When news stories reported on statistics of the epidemic, whether national or regional, they often discussed the consequences related to chronic pain patients and/or the treatment of pain. For instance, articles reported how "current policies to limit opioid prescriptions leave some pain patients high and dry, resulting in a new wave of unintended consequences for patients with untreated chronic pain," as well as how "the rush to deal with the nation's opioid crisis is making life much harder for people with chronic pain ... [patients need] these pain meds to function" (Featherstone 2018; Janke 2019). Similarly, we identified the consequence frame in articles that offered statistical overviews about the epidemic, regionally or nationally, related to crime, doctors, and effects since prescribing guidelines were adjusted.

5.3.2 *The Strategy Frame*

The *strategy* frame (n = 180, 36.6%) appeared when newspapers emphasized initiatives being undertaken to combat the opioid epidemic and/or mitigating chronic pain. Of note, the CDC authored the "Guidelines for Prescribing Opioids for Chronic Pain" in 2016 (CDC 2016). The guidelines were published in a misguided effort to curb legal opioid prescribing and reduce overdose deaths, and this action received substantial coverage in U.S. newspapers. However, most opioid overdose deaths have been driven by illicit (i.e., illegally obtained) heroin and fentanyl since 2010 (CDC 2025). The guidelines were intended to be narrowly applied as guidance for primary care providers prescribing opioids for long-term chronic pain management. The guidelines suggested daily dosage limits on opioids, as well as recommended consensual deprescribing (i.e., working alongside patients to slowly reduce the dose of their prescription opioid medication) without adequate alternative non-opioid pain relief medications or therapies being available or covered by insurance for most chronic pain patients. Yet, the guidelines became widely misapplied. As a result, chronic pain patients were forced to rapidly taper down their legally prescribed opioids, leading to widespread suicides and use of illicit drugs among these patients (Agnoli et al. 2021; Hintz and Applequist 2025). As one article summarized, "When the [CDC] introduced guidelines for opioid prescribing in 2016, doctors began treating pain patients differently. It didn't matter if a patient had been stable and benefiting from [opioid] medication for many years [,] doctors pulled back" (Anne Fuqua 2018). These guidelines were active from 2016 until they were replaced with new guidelines in 2022 developed in partnership with chronic pain patients and advocates (CDC 2022).

In addition to covering the 2016 CDC guidelines, newspaper articles adopting the strategy frame also devoted significant discussion to the potential for prescribers to leverage emerging non-opioid pain management options. Many articles discussed opioids as one type of pain management to be utilized selectively alongside other complementary and alternative non-opioid therapies. As one article explains, "[Expert] describes pain as a car with four flat tires. One medication or treatment only puts air in one of the wheels, she says; the other three can be filled up with tools like physical therapy, counseling, goal-setting, acupuncture, and more" (Roubein 2018). Medical marijuana was discussed as another potential strategic solution to the opioid crisis. As one article discussing the need for more clinicians to join experimental chronic pain medical marijuana programs explained, "For some of the patients I have seen, suffering from chronic pain or seizures, there is a big hope for them that the quality of life could improve through medical marijuana" (Schmitt 2018). An article published later in the sample window reflected on the efficacy of medical marijuana for reducing opioid abuse, "With the spread of medical marijuana and its effectiveness in treating chronic pain, many medical conditions that lead to painkiller prescriptions can now be treated through this alternate system, rather than sending patients down the path of potential addiction" (Sewell 2018). Medical marijuana was already legal in 17 U.S. states prior to 2012, and by 2022 most U.S. states had legalized or decriminalized some form of medical marijuana (DISA 2025). Hence, articles employing the strategy frame reflected shifting initiatives intended to curb the opioid crisis.

5.3.3 *The Culpability Frame*

The *culpability* frame (n = 105, 21.3%) appeared when newspaper articles focused on the legal actions taken against specific entities deemed to be at fault for the opioid epidemic. These legal actions often centered on pharmaceutical companies manufacturing medications taken by chronic pain patients. A variety of individuals, groups, and organizations were deemed culpable for the opioid crisis by U.S. newspapers. Covering legal proceedings, U.S. newspapers reported on the alleged wrongdoings of (and lawsuits and settlements against) the Sackler family, pharmaceutical companies such as Purdue Pharmaceuticals, and other health care organizations. Providing a final update on a lawsuit against Johnson & Johnson, one newspaper article summarized, "Following a seven-week trial…Balkman ruled Johnson & Johnson…helped fuel the opioid crisis with an aggressive and misleading marketing campaign that overstated how effective the drugs were for treating chronic pain and understated the risk of addiction" (Associated Press 2019). This quotation was cited by reports from various news outlets in 2019. Other newspaper articles focused on the comments of litigators about their satisfaction with judgments against pharmaceutical companies. For instance, one article reported on comments made to Judge Michael Ramsey Scott by Washington Attorney General Bob Ferguson following a successful settlement against three pharmaceutical companies:

> These companies knew what would happen if they failed to meet their duties… We know they were aware of the harms flowing from their conduct because in private correspondence, company executives mocked individuals suffering the painful effects of opioid dependence… They displayed a callous disregard for the communities and people who bear the impact of their greed. (Johnson 2021)

In sum, newspaper articles framed chronic pain as a site of culpability by making attributions of responsibility to various entities based on legal proceedings. These articles function to keep readers abreast of ongoing legal proceedings while simultaneously reiterating comments supporting successful litigation regarding the opioid crisis to the public.

5.3.4 The Human-Interest Frame

Finally, the *human-interest* frame ($n = 61$, 12.4%) appeared when newspaper articles highlighted the stories of chronic pain patients whose lives were negatively affected by opioid manufacturing and prescribing policies intended to mitigate the opioid crisis. Some articles highlighted the harms of nonconsensual opioid deprescribing on chronic pain patients, for example:

> My opioid crisis is wondering whether each time I fill my medications will be the last time. I wonder how much longer I'll be able to do the things I enjoy. I'm 38 years old. There's so much that I want to do with my life. I want to go back to work part time, but I'm afraid to, because my future is so uncertain. I feel like I'm on death row. (Fuqua 2018)

Other articles amplified chronic pain patients' frustrations with how opioid prescribing policies interfered with their ability to access their medications. For example, one patient explained, "Might this dependence lead to addiction? At 84, I don't care… before I would… suffer unbearably… I would die by suicide. I hope those who control patients' access to opiates… continue providing pain relief to those who need it badly" (Readers

2022). Likewise, another patient noted, "I was on long-term opiate therapy for 12 years. Before my involuntary taper… I was a fully engaged wife, mother and caregiver… Pain is a cancer that has consumed my life with grinding, bedridden indolence." Human-interest newspaper stories highlighted the perspectives of chronic pain patients who became collateral damage in the war on opioids.

In sum, four dominant frames characterized U.S. newspaper coverage of chronic pain in relation to the opioid epidemic from 2012 to 2022. These frames underscored the impacts of the opioid epidemic on chronic pain patients and/or the treatment of pain (n = 146, 29.7%), outlined strategies for combating the epidemic and/or mitigating chronic pain (n = 180, 36.6%), relayed legal and moral ascriptions of culpability for the epidemic (n = 105, 21.3%), and highlighted chronic pain patients' perspectives (n = 61, 12.4%).

5.4 Characters in Newspaper Coverage of Chronic Pain in Relation to the Opioid Crisis

Major characters represented included (a) chronic pain patients, (b) pharmaceutical companies responsible for producing opioid pain medications, (c) U.S. government officials including Presidents, (d) major health organizations including the CDC, National Institutes of Health (NIH), the U.S. Food and Drug Administration (FDA), American Medical Association (AMA), and National Institute on Drug Abuse (NIDA), (e) law enforcement including police officers, the Department of Justice (DOJ), and Drug Enforcement Agency (DEA) among others, and (f) celebrities including Prince (who died of an opioid overdose).

5.4.1 Chronic Pain Patients

A first major character type present in the articles in the final sample was chronic pain patients. Oftentimes, chronic pain patients were treated as a monolith in news coverage of the opioid crisis, where their perspectives were often lost in the coverage. When chronic pain patients were discussed explicitly as a central focus of a news story, they were often characterized as collateral damage in the war on opioids (e.g., "'one-size-fits-all' solutions… do nothing except disenfranchise chronic pain sufferers"; Maxwell 2019). As one article pointed out, "[Chronic pain patients] take [opioids] to be able to participate in life and addicts take it to escape from life. Without the medication [chronic pain patients] don't have quality of life" (Borchert 2019). Another article also explained, "It is essential to eliminate stigma from the conversation about the opioid crisis and ensure that our policies do not place undue burden on... Americans who have... chronic pain, many of whom are appropriately prescribed opioids" (Featherstone 2018). Moreover, the sampled news articles noted that the 2016 CDC's opioid medication prescribing guidelines had caused harmful consequences for chronic pain patients. For example, some chronic pain patients were forced to turn to illicit street drugs in lieu of legally prescribed medications to manage their pain, leading to increased rates of overdoses and deaths as well as mental health crisis events (Janke 2019; Agnoli et al. 2021).

This undue burden placed on chronic pain patients due to policies intended to curb opioid prescribing came at the risk of legal interference from federal and state enforcement agencies, such as the DEA. One headline illustrating this point read, "Chronic pain patients suffer in opioid crisis as doctors fear retribution" (St. Amour 2019). Clinicians prescribing opioids became targets of "raids" by the DEA and other enforcement authorities. Clinicians were also threatened with formal medical complaints, incarceration, and sometimes the loss of medical licensure. These threats often left chronic pain patients without access to their needed medications by creating a chilling effect on opioid prescribing for other clinicians. Another article told the story of a chronic pain patient named David Lackey who, following a long career as a machinist, suffered from arthritis and degenerative disc disease. David's clinician was raided by the DEA, as the article explains:

> [David] had an appointment scheduled the following week after the raid but soon found himself without the medication he had regularly taken or any records to give to another doctor... there were no referrals or contingency plans for patients who would soon find themselves without pain medication. (Borchert 2019)

Later in the article, we learn that David endured a painful withdrawal after losing access to his prescribed opioid medications and died of a heart attack two months after the raid had occurred. Stories like those of David Lackey illustrate how chronic pain patients become acceptable collateral damage in the war on opioids.

We would be remiss not to mention that this undue burden does not fall equally onto all chronic pain patients. Evaluations of chronic pain patients' pain and credibility are affected by numerous biases, including sexism and racism. Female patients, for example, are less likely to be believed when expressing pain to a clinician and are less likely to be offered sufficient pain medication and more likely to be directed to psychological care when compared to male patients (Guzikevits et al. 2024). White clinicians often hold inaccurate stereotypes purporting that Black, Indigenous, and people of color (BIPOC) with chronic pain feel less pain than white patients (Hoffman et al. 2016, 4296–4301). One BIPOC female patient explained her perspective on the relationship between gender, race, and pain management:

> We have research that shows that gender and race play a huge part in how people get access and how they perceive people being 'whiny' and drug seeking... It's not far-fetched to be a 10 [on a pain scale] - and what happens when you are a 10 and you are a woman of color or a minority and you're asking a provider? The default is that you are a drug seeker and you're being whiny and that you're being dramatic, and those words are often being thrown around in doctors' offices I am in. (Lee 2019)

In addition to sexism and racism, classism also plays a role in clinicians' evaluation of patients' pain. For instance, female BIPOC chronic pain patients from lower socioeconomic backgrounds are more likely to be accused of malingering, or faking pain to receive a secondary benefit such as pain medication, attention, or disability benefits (Pryma 2017, 66–73.) These patients accused of malingering are often mistakenly characterized as "pill shopping opioid junkies" by clinicians and other health care providers (St. Amour 2019). As one chronic pain patient lamented, "Frankly, when you're dealing with that much pain, you can look pretty desperate, but that doesn't mean that you're struggling with a substance abuse disorder" (St. Amour, 2019). Multiple minoritized chronic pain patients must manage the undue burden of chronic pain caused by rapidly shifting opioid prescribing policies, but they must also manage the stress of encountering various biases in health care settings. As one author reported, "Beyond living with untreated pain, patients suffer from the stress of encountering racism and implicit bias in health-care settings. Stress can literally 'get under the skin,' causing harmful changes in the body that over time contribute to poor health" (Khatri 2019). These intersecting sites of oppression influence both how chronic pain patients (and their pain) are regarded and the quality and amount of health care they receive, and eventually their overall health.

5.4.1.1 Specific Characterizations of Chronic Pain (Patients)

The preceding section reports on the overall portrayal of chronic pain patients within news coverage of the opioid crisis in the past decade. In addition to discussing chronic pain patients broadly, many articles also elevated specific caricatures of chronic pain patients by highlighting certain narrow characteristics. These characteristics included the occupation of the chronic pain patients (e.g., athlete, laborer, and Veteran) as well as ascribed behavioral stereotypes (e.g., drug addict, "doctor shopper," criminal, and victim of suicide). We unpack these caricatures below, and in doing so, illustrate the (lack of) representativeness of pain patients in news coverage of the opioid crisis.

Regarding chronic pain patients' occupations, patients were primarily characterized as former athletes, veterans suffering from service-related injuries and ailments, and laborers who have (like David Lackey in our sample above) accrued chronic pain over the course of their careers. One article detailed traditional manufacturing jobs in Rust Belt towns, painting a distinct picture of such laborers and their opioid use:

> All that remains is an entire generation of Americans whose agency has been fundamentally altered, their sense of purpose eroded by perpetual joblessness and the possession of skills no longer in demand. Their bodies, ravaged by chronic pain resulting from years of manual labor, received second-rate care through underfunded Veterans Affairs, Medicare and Medicaid programs staffed with physicians who sought to cure persistent pain through indefinite opioid use. Once locals had become addicted, the increased demand for prescriptions was met by for-profit "pill mills" willing to write a script for anyone with a pulse, operated by the sleaziest of medical practitioners. (Ribel 2016)

As displayed, beyond characterizing chronic pain patients in terms of their current or former occupations, chronic pain patients were ascribed stereotypes related to their behavior and disposition. First, chronic pain patients were characterized in news coverage of the opioid crisis as alleged or potential future drug addicts. As one article lamenting the state of Massachusetts' reticence to adopt the 2016 CDC guidelines noted, "The state hasn't adopted the CDC Chronic Pain Guidelines regarding opiate prescriptions, which reduce the risk of addiction for chronic pain patients" (Webb 2018). This article seems to inadvertently attribute addiction to legal opioid prescriptions written for chronic pain patients. Another article made a similar conflation, beginning by reporting on "Floyd and his girlfriend...who were prescribed opioids for chronic back and neck pain" and then immediately discussing opioid abuse, addiction, and patients' use of illicit street drugs including heroin (Wang 2021). These examples illustrate how chronic pain patients become (sometimes implicitly) associated with opioid addiction, misuse, and abuse.

Second, chronic pain patients were characterized as "doctor shoppers," a label ascribed to patients who see numerous clinicians for their illness(es) for a nefarious purpose such as receiving a prescribed opioid medication (Hintz et al. 2018). One article detailed how technology is used during the prescription process in an attempt to curb this practice: "If a controlled substance is prescribed, the database tracks the drug, the doctor and the patient by date of birth ... the computer then looks for patterns. It is designed to reduce excessive prescription refills and doctor shopping" (Moore 2016). The tracking system was said to make it "easy to detect 'doctor shoppers'... when a person goes from doctor to doctor looking for an excessive amount of a certain prescribed medication or treatment after being told 'no' by previous doctors" (Fair 2016).

Third, chronic pain patients were characterized as criminals engaging in illegal activity. For instance, when reporting on the impacts of forced tapering, newspaper articles often suggested the likelihood of chronic pain patients seeking medication illegally: "Forcing pain patients to reduce their dose of opioids or not allowing a prescriber to give a patient the dose that they need, leads to suffering, to pain patients searching for illicit and more dangerous alternatives" (No Author 2019). Other illegal activities were also mentioned in relation to chronic pain patients. As one article reported, "Judge Hanley noted that many of the retail thefts, burglaries, car break-ins and simple assaults he heard are also driven by heroin. 'The [prescription opioid] pills lead to the heroin, and it just destroys people.'" (Lord 2016).

Finally, chronic pain patients were associated with suicides and suicidality. Forced tapering results in dramatic increases in rates of suicide for chronic pain patients. Drawing this connection in news coverage served both to highlight a problem resulting from curbing legal opioid prescriptions and to perpetuate the stereotype that chronic pain patients suffer from mental illnesses (Agnoli et al. 2021; Hintz and Applequist 2025). One article summarized, “Serious chronic pain… it leads to depression. It leads to suicide. People can’t take care of their own basic functions…” (Murphy 2019). Other articles positioned suicide as a rational option for chronic pain patients deprived of access to prescription opioids, noting, “[Chronic pain patients] are tortured by their pain, and they often see suicide as a means of escape… suicides in the U.S. continue to climb… people with chronic pain are at least twice as likely to report suicidal behaviors” (Webster 2021). This view of suicide as a rational option continued as news coverage began to focus on the barriers that chronic pain patients faced in accessing opioid medications following the implementation of the 2016 opioid prescribing guidelines. An article recounted one male pain patient’s struggle:

> [Patient] cannot receive any of his medication and is instead forced to visit his pharmacy the exact day that his prescription runs out. In the event of the pharmacy being out of stock, [he] could be forced to live without his medication for as long as it takes the pharmacy to restock. This would be bad for any chronic pain sufferer, as [he] said, ‘There are patients whose pain is so bad that they’re suicidal, and they’ll have no effective treatment beyond opioids. They’re fast, they’re effective, and they’re cheap.’ (Craig 2019)

In sum, chronic pain patients appeared as prominent characters across the sample. Although many articles only discussed chronic pain patients broadly or as a monolith, when more nuanced discussion occurred, these patients were characterized in terms of their current or former occupations and (alleged) ascribed behaviors.

5.4.2 *Pharmaceutical Companies*

Pharmaceutical companies were a second prominent character type represented across the sample. Although numerous pharmaceutical companies appeared throughout the sample, Purdue Pharmaceuticals (an exclusive manufacturer of opioids and the manufacturer of the notorious OxyContin) became the target of significant public scrutiny, as was discussed above in the culpability frame section. We offer additional exemplars illustrating how pharmaceutical companies appeared as characters later in this chapter (see the section on legal events).

5.4.3 *U.S. Government Officials*

Articles included in the final sample third offered coverage and critiques of actions taken by U.S. government officials such as presidents (i.e., Barack Obama, Donald Trump, and Joe Biden) and governors. The declaration of the opioid crisis as a national emergency garnered substantial news media coverage, as one article reported, "President Donald Trump has declared the opioid crisis a national public health emergency but stopped short…of declaring a state of emergency that would've given states access to funding from the federal Disaster Relief Fund." Another article detailed a visit to Haywood County, North Carolina from Governor Roy Cooper:

> We wanted to come to Haywood County, number one because we know this is an acute problem here, but also the innovative ways this county is attacking this problem… I know that treatment requires, in many instances, more and better healthcare coverage… one of my missions is to close the healthcare coverage gap here … and across our state.

Government officials were coded upon any mention, aiding in the contextualization of this epidemic across news coverage. Such mentions ranged from critique of U.S. officials to detailed efforts officials undertook to mend circumstances in particular geographical regions and/or the country writ large.

5.4.4 *Major Health Organizations*

Related to, yet distinct from, U.S. government officials is our fourth character type—major health organizations. Major U.S. health organizations relevant to the opioid crisis were featured substantially in news publications, such as the NIH, CDC, and FDA. The FDA was particularly criticized for approving opioids for the treatment of chronic non-cancer pain. In a review of the book *Dopesick* (also the subject of a Hulu show), one article narrated, "By the first decade of the new century, any doctor in any small town, under the dispensation of a new FDA-approved prescription, could suddenly provide opioids to people with low back issues" (Okie 2018). Purdue Pharma also used the cover of FDA approval to usurp accountability for the unchecked proliferation of opioid use for chronic pain, writing, "As a matter of law Purdue's statements are not false or misleading… The medications at issue are FDA-approved to treat chronic noncancer pain... statements consistent with that approval cannot be deceptive or fraudulent as a matter of law" (Okie 2018). News articles also included coverage of efforts enacted by major health organizations (such as the CDC) to curb opioid prescribing, "Guidelines such as those written by the CDC... hope to reduce the availability of prescription opioids as one solution to combat the epidemic" (Janke 2019). Thus, major health organizations were prominent news characters.

5.4.5 *Law Enforcement*

Law enforcement organizations and officers were a fifth character type appearing across the sample. One article detailed the need for police officers to administer Narcan (i.e., a medication used to reverse the effects of opioids) to treat overdoses in emergencies, which requires the sheriff's department to carry the drug alongside an ambulance: "Police officers aren't doctors, they'd be administering a medicine... It's a huge, huge shift" (Dolmage 2017). State officials also became involved in federal lawsuits, as reported on in local newspapers, "State Attorney General Ellen Rosenblum join[ed] 47 other states and the District of Columbia in suing Purdue [Pharma] and other companies involved in the fraudulent promotion of painkillers" (Shinn 2021). Law enforcement officials were essential in news coverage of the opioid crisis.

5.4.6 *Prince*

Finally, celebrities, specifically the singer Prince, appeared prominently in the sample. As one headline summarizes, "Opioid epidemic claims Prince as most famous victim" (Gensler 2016). Prince died in April 2016 due to an accidental overdose of fentanyl, an opioid medication. The popstar was repeatedly referenced in relation to accidental overdose, putting a "national spotlight on the issue" (Stewart 2016). Stories tended to call into question Prince's doctor and his management (or mismanagement) of Prince's pain.

In sum, news publications prominently featured several characters relevant to discussions of chronic pain in relation to the opioid crisis. These characters included chronic pain patients, pharmaceutical companies, U.S. government officials, major health organizations, law enforcement, and celebrities.

5.5 Significant Events in Newspaper Coverage of Chronic Pain in Relation to the Opioid Crisis

Finally, in addition to coding for the dominant frames adopted by newspaper coverage of chronic pain (patients) in relationship to the opioid crisis, as well as characters present in such coverage, we also coded for the *significant events*, or the broader events utilized to discuss chronic pain (patients) in relationship to the opioid crisis. The significant events highlighted included (a) changes or implementation of policies regarding opioid prescribing, (b) legal events such as ongoing civil and criminal litigation, (c) the COVID-19 pandemic, as well as (d) the appearance of popular media portrayals of the opioid crisis (e.g., *Dopesick*) (Piqué-Buisan et al. 2024).

5.5.1 Policy Events

First, the articles in the final sample referred to proposed or instated policies related to opioid prescribing and pain management. These articles distinctly encompassed treatment-oriented policies, such as the Intractable Pain Act, the FDA's approval of OxyContin, and changes to the CDC's prescribing guidelines. Some headlines of the articles covering policy events include "New CDC Guidelines Seen as Boost for Chiropractic Care" and "CDC Issues New Guidance on Prescribed Opioids for Pain" (Piqué-Buisan et al. 2024).

5.5.2 Legal Events

Second, the articles included in the sample referred to significant legal events concerning the opioid crisis. For instance, news articles highlighted litigation against Purdue Pharma, the manufacturer of OxyContin, as well as their responses to legal charges of wrongdoing. As one article summarized, "The lawsuit... claimed Purdue Pharma spurred the opioid epidemic through an aggressive and successful marketing campaign designed to persuade prescribers and patients that opioids can and should be used for chronic pain" (Williams 2019). Another article reported Purdue Pharma's response, being that it "vigorously denies the allegations filed... and will continue to defend itself against these misleading attacks" (Joanna Walters 2019). Events related to lawsuits, court cases, judicial decisions, and legal actions were coded as legal events (Mulvihill and Seewer 2022).

5.5.3 *COVID-19*

Given that the data collection period for this study ended in December 2022, newspaper articles drawing parallels between the opioid crisis and the COVID-19 pandemic were prevalent in the sample. For instance, "Blose refers to the COVID-19 pandemic and opioid epidemic as a syndemic, a network of health problems that have common underpinnings and exploit existing disparities and underlying health conditions" (Shinn 2021). Some articles underscored the relationship between orders to social distance, limit travel, and staying at home and the opioid crisis: "The thing that would save thousands of lives from COVID-19 was the same thing that would kill hundreds from an overdose" (Leal 2021).

5.5.4 *Media Events*

Numerous books, journalistic exposés, videos, movies, and television shows have been made about the opioid epidemic and the treatment of chronic pain in the U.S., which became significant media events. These included popular shows/portrayals of the opioid epidemic such as "*Dopesick*" and "*Crime of the Century.*" For instance, the article "High on money '*Dopesick*' rips pharma fam & pill pushers" discussed portrayals of the opioid epidemic and pharmaceutical companies' marketing techniques: "The pills flow down, from Richard Sackler (Michael Stuhlbarg) to the pharmaceutical reps (Will Poulter and Phillipa Soo) to the doctors (Michael Keaton) to the pain patients (Kaitlyn Dever). The lie flows in that same direction: 'OxyContin is nonaddictive'" (Feldman 2021).

In sum, we coded significant events in articles discussing chronic pain (patients) in relation to the health policy, ongoing litigation, the COVID-19 pandemic, and media portrayals of the opioid crisis.

5.6 Conclusion

Now that we have reviewed the dominant frames, characters, and significant events present in newspaper coverage of chronic pain (patients) in relation to the opioid epidemic, we conclude this chapter with suggestions for how media outlets can improve their reporting on and representation of chronic pain (patients) when communicating about the opioid crisis. Of most importance, our analysis revealed that news stories often either fail to discuss chronic pain patients specifically, or when doing so, perpetuate potentially harmful stereotypes about them. These findings also revealed how chronic pain patients have been marginalized in news coverage concerning the opioid crisis. Media outlets must take care when discussing the issue of chronic pain to humanize these patients and discuss issues affecting chronic pain patients with nuance and sensitivity. Human-interest articles were the least represented frame type across the sample. Therefore, for example, rather than broad brushing all chronic pain patients with stereotypes about substance use, news outlets could highlight these human-interest stories that capture the nuances of chronic pain patients needing pain relief while simultaneously balancing shifting opioid prescribing practices.

We noticed that often the proximity of certain claims (e.g., introducing chronic pain into a piece of journalism, then quickly pivoting to discuss heroin overdoses) might negatively affect the general public's perceptions of chronic pain patients (e.g., as users of heroin or other illicit drugs). Specifically, when reporting on the opioid epidemic, journalists should be aware of and acknowledge: (a) the negative and often deadly consequences that result(ed) from policies requiring the forced tapering of chronic pain patients' opioid prescriptions, as well as (b) the utility of opioids for chronic pain, leading to life-changing outcomes (e.g., enhanced quality of life, increased physical ability, and reduced depression), often and likely without the accompaniment of substance use disorder.

We also want to acknowledge the realities of substance use disorder and its relationship to the opioid epidemic and chronic pain. Both chronic pain patients and individuals with substance use disorder are stigmatized in coverage of the opioid epidemic. People experiencing addiction are often mistakenly depicted as selfish, shameful, and curable, when in reality addiction might be better understood as an incurable disease that is impacted by environmental, situational, and relational factors (Wolfe and Scharp 2022). It is our intention to highlight the fact that, although chronic pain and substance abuse can certainly co-occur, they are not synonymous. All chronic pain patients are not current or future victims of substance use disorder; just as someone with substance use disorder is not assumed to have chronic pain. However, media coverage often intertwines and conflates these two overlapping yet distinct health experiences. We encourage media outlets to be more cognizant of the presence of such assumptions, as well as stereotypes, within their published work, which often perpetuate harms for both chronic pain patients and the millions of individuals in the U.S. battling substance use disorder.

This chapter was written with the intention to contextualize overly simplistic understandings of the opioid epidemic, and in doing so amplify the voices of chronic pain patients who have been harmed in efforts to ameliorate the opioid crisis. How media outlets communicate about and depict chronic pain patients and the opioid epidemic plays an integral role in shaping public perceptions of this topic. Therefore, media depictions should do more to humanize this issue by focusing on the people in these stories rather than forwarding often problematic and stigmatizing portrayals. The attitudes cultivated and reinforced by the media then become sedimented in policies reforming the provision of opioids, as well as clinicians' practice of healthcare. We hope that this chapter empowers communicators and practitioners with the knowledge to improve how chronic pain (patients) are viewed in relation to the opioid crisis.

References

Agnoli, Alicia, Guibo Xing, Daniel J. Tancredi, Elizabeth Magnan, Anthony Jerant, and Joshua J. Fenton. 2021. Association of Dose Tapering with Overdose or Mental Health Crisis among Patients Prescribed Long-Term Opioids. *JAMA* 326 (5): 411–419. https://doi.org/10.1001/jama.2021.11013.

Borchert, Courtney. 2019. *Pain Patients Become Collateral Damage in Opioid Crisis*. Odessa, TX: Odessa American.

Centers for Disease Control and Prevention. 2016. *CDC Guideline for Prescribing Opioids for Chronic Pain—United States*. https://www.cdc.gov/mmwr/volumes/65/rr/rr6501e1.htm.

Centers for Disease Control and Prevention. 2022. *CDC Clinical Practice Guideline for Prescribing Opioids for Pain—United States*. https://pubmed.ncbi.nlm.nih.gov/36327391/.

Centers for Disease Control and Prevention. 2025. *Understanding the Opioid Overdose Epidemic*. https://www.cdc.gov/overdose-prevention/about/understanding-the-opioid-overdose-epidemic.html.

DISA. 2025. *Marijuana Legality by State*. https://disa.com/marijuana-legality-by-state-old/.

Dolmage, David. 2017. Substance Abuse Coalition Defines Legislative Priorities. *Newton Daily News* (Iowa).

Entman, Robert M. 1993. Framing: Toward Clarification of a Fractured Paradigm. *Journal of Communication* 43 (4): 51–58.

Fair, Julia. 2016. New Prescription Guidelines Set in Hopes of Diminishing Number of Opiate Overdoses in Ohio. *The Post*, February 9. https://www.

thepostathens.com/article/2016/02/new-prescription-guidelines-set-in-hopes-of-diminishing-number-of-opiate-overdoses-in-ohio.

Featherstone, Charles H. 2018. *Pain Patients Caught in Crossfire of Drug War.* Columbia Basin Herald.

Feldman, Kate. 2021. High on Money: 'Dopesick' Rips Pharma Fam & Pill Pushers. *Daily News* (New York).

Fuqua, Anne. 2018. The Other Opioid Crisis: Inability to Manage Pain. *Dayton Daily News* (Ohio).

Gensler, Howard. 2016. Opioid Epidemic Claims Prince as Most Famous Victim. *The Philadelphia Daily News.*

Giles, David, and Rachel L. Shaw. 2009. The Psychology of News Influence and the Development of Media Framing Analysis. *Social and Personality Psychology Compass* 3 (4): 375–393. https://doi.org/10.1111/j.1751-9004.2009.00180.x.

Gunning, Jacqueline N., Lili R. Romann, and Elizabeth A. Hintz. 2024. Framing Chronic Pain in U.S. News Coverage of the Opioid Epidemic (2012–2022). *Health Communication* 39 (13): 3122–3133. https://doi.org/10.1080/10410236.2024.2304494.

Guzikevits, Mika, Tom Gordon-Hecker, David Rekhtman, and Shoham Choshen-Hillel. 2024. Sex Bias in Pain Management Decisions. *Proceedings of the National Academy of Sciences* 121 (33): e2401331121. https://doi.org/10.1073/pnas.2401331121.

Hayes, Andrew F, and Klaus Krippendorff. 2007. Answering the call for a standard reliability measure for coding data. *Communication Methods and Measures 1 (1): 77–89.*

Hintz, Elizabeth A., and Janelle Applequist. 2025. 'Saving Us to Death': Ideology and Communicative (Dis)enfranchisement in Misapplications of the 2016 CDC Opioid Prescribing Guidelines. *Health Communication* 40 (4): 702–712. https://doi.org/10.1080/10410236.2024.2363674.

Hoffman, Kelly M., Sophie Trawalter, Jordan R. Axt, and M. Norman Oliver. 2016. Racial Bias in Pain Assessment and Treatment Recommendations, and False Beliefs About Biological Differences Between Blacks and Whites. *Proceedings of the National Academy of Sciences 113 (16): 4296–4301.* https://doi.org/10.1073/pnas.1516047113.

International Association for the Study of Pain. 2024. *Terminology.* https://www.iasp-pain.org/resources/terminology/.

Janke, Aaron. "The Opioid Crisis, Chronic Pain, and Insurance Coverage." The Philadelphia Inquirer, January 11, 2019. https://www.inquirer.com/opinion/commentary/opioid-crisis-chronic-pain-insurance-coverage-20190111.html.

Johnson, Gene. 2021. Washington Seeks Over $38 Billion from Opioid Distributors. *Telegraph Herald* (Dubuque, IA), November 15. https://www.

heraldnet.com/northwest/washington-seeks-over-38-billion-from-opioid-distributors/.
Khatri, Uché Blackstock. "The Opioid Crisis Reveals Racism in Health Care and Access to Buprenorphine." The Philadelphia Inquirer, December 23, 2019. https://www.inquirer.com/health/expert-opinions/opioid-crisis-racism-healthcare-buprenorphine-20191223.html.
Krippendorff, Klaus. 2018. *Content Analysis: An Introduction to Its Methodology*. Sage Publications.
Leal, Sofia. 2021. How Covid-19 Impacted the Opioid Crisis in Chicago. *The DePaulia*, May 23. https://depauliaonline.com/54045/focus/how-covid-19-impacted-the-opioid-crisis-in-chicago/.
Lee, Jasmin. 2019. Panelists Examines Opioid Criminalization, Medical Access. *The Michigan Daily*, October 3. https://www.michigandaily.com/news/science/panelists-examines-opioid-criminalization-medical-access/.
Lord, Rich. 2016. One Day in the Opioid Epidemic: Experience 24 Hours of Addiction to See What the Pittsburgh Region Is Facing. *Pittsburgh Post-Gazette*.
Matthias, Marianne S., Tasneem L. Talib, and Monica A. Huffman. 2020. Managing Chronic Pain in an Opioid Crisis: What Is the Role of Shared Decision-Making? *Health Communication* 35 (10): 1239–1247. https://doi.org/10.1080/10410236.2019.1625000.
Maxwell Craig, 2019. The US is mishandling the opioid epidemic The Lawrentian: Lawrence University.
Moore, William. 2016. Authorities Deal with Opioid Epidemic. *Northeast Mississippi Daily Journal*, Tupelo.
Mulvihill, Geoff, and John Seewer. 2022. Purdue Pharma, States OK Opioid Settlement. *Chicago Daily Herald*, March 3. https://www.ems1.com/opioids/articles/purdue-pharma-us-states-agree-to-new-opioid-settlement-s0EndCFt2UN7cbp0/.
Murphy. "Oklahoma Attorney Blames Corporate Greed for Opioid Crisis." AP News, May 28, 2019. https://apnews.com/general-news-616ef7ba545e4e5287e406182126938d.
Neuendorff, Kimberly A. 2011. Content Analysis–A Methodological Primer for Gender Research. *Sex Roles* 64 (1): 276–289. https://doi.org/10.1007/s11199-010-9893-0.
No Author. 2019. Forcing Treatment and Tying the Hands of Physicians Won't Solve the Opioid Crisis. *The Philadelphia Inquirer (Opinion)*, April 8. https://www.inquirer.com/opinion/editorials/prescription-limits-opioid-coerced-treatment-pennsylvania-harrisburg-20190408.html.
Okie, Susan. 2018. Book Review: 'Dopesick': Heartbreaking Stories of Young Lives Lost, Families Crushed in the Opioid Epidemic. *Chicago Daily Herald*, October 8. https://www.dailyherald.com/20181006/lifestyle/book-review-

dopesick-heartbreaking-stories-of-young-lives-lost-families-crushed-in-the-opioid-e/.

Piqué-Buisan, Joel, Josep-E. Baños, and Irene Cambra-Badii. 2024. Telling the Story of the Opioid Crisis: A Narrative Analysis of the TV Series Dopesick. *PLOS ONE* 19 (4): e0301681. https://doi.org/10.1371/journal.pone.0301681.

Pryma, Jane. 2017. "Even My Sister Says I'm Acting Like a Crazy to Get a Check": Race, Gender, and Moral Boundary-Work in Women's Claims of Disabling Chronic Pain. *Social Science & Medicine* 181:66–73. https://doi.org/10.1016/j.socscimed.2017.03.048.

Readers. 2022. Opioids, Chronic Pain and Addiction Letters. *The New York Times*, March 22. https://www.nytimes.com/2022/03/22/opinion/letters/opioids-chronic-pain-addiction.html.

Ribel, Matthew. 2016. The Opiate Crisis Is 2016's Most Underrated Campaign Issue. *Emory Wheel*, September 14. https://www.emorywheel.com/article/2016/09/the-opiate-crisis-is-2016s-most-underrated-campaign-issue.

Roubein, Rachel. 2018. *Sessions Triggers Pain Debate with Opioids Remarks.* The Hill.

Schmitt, Ben. 2018. Pennsylvania Seeks More Doctors to Join Medical Pot Program. *TribLive*, February 11. https://archive.triblive.com/local/westmoreland/pennsylvania-seeks-more-doctors-to-join-medical-pot-program.

Sewell, Dan. 2018. Boehner, Weld Hired to Promote Legal Pot. *Charleston Gazette-Mail.*

Shinn, Sara. "Benton County Drug Court Celebrates Successes While Confronting Ongoing Opioid Challenges." Corvallis Gazette-Times, June 25, 2021. https://gazettetimes.com/news/local/article_d5664468-dbe6-51af-bb53-1ddfe3106ec4.html.

St. Amour, Madeline. 2019. Chronic Pain Patients Suffer in Opioid Crisis as Doctors Fear Retribution. *Daily Camera*, June 2. https://www.dailycamera.com/2019/06/02/chronic-pain-patients-suffer-in-opioid-crisis-as-doctors-fear-retribution.

Stanton, Marsha. 2017. Don't Forget the Chronic Pain Sufferer. *Deseret Morning News* Salt Lake City.

Stewart, Chris. 2016 = Pill-abuse problem in Ohio overlooked Death of music icon Prince has put national spotlight on issue. In-Depth coverage local impact. Dayton Daily News (Ohio).

Vos, Theo, Christine Allen, Megha Arora, et al. 2016. Global, Regional, and National Incidence, Prevalence, and Years Lived with Disability for 310 Diseases and Injuries, 1990–2015: A Systematic Analysis for the Global Burden of Disease Study 2015. *The Lancet* 388 (10053): 1545–1602. https://doi.org/10.1016/S0140-6736(16)31678-6.

Walters, Joanna. 2019. Purdue Pharma: OxyContin Maker Faces Lawsuits from Nearly Every US State. *The Guardian*, June 4. https://www.theguardian.

com/us-news/2019/jun/03/purdue-opioids-lawsuit-oxycontin-california-maine-hawaii.

Wang, Renee. 2021. How Divergent Narratives of Opioid Drug Addictions Create Lives of Expectation and Exception. *The California Aggie: University of California*, Davis.

Webb, Kaila. 2018. A Wealth of Data: A Map of the Massachusetts Opioid Epidemic. *Pioneer Institute for Public Policy Research.* https://pioneerinstitute.org/category/blog/blog-healthcare/blog-healthcare-transparency.

Webster, Lynn. 2021. Trading One Crisis for Another Is No Answer to the Opioid Epidemic. *The Salt Lake Tribune*, May 20. https://www.sltrib.com/opinion/commentary/2021/05/20/lynn-webster-trading-one/.

Williams 2019. State's lawsuit against opioid producer dismissed by judge, The Bismarck Tribune Tess Williams.

Wolfe, Brooke H., and Kristina M. Scharp. 2022. An (In)curable Disease? Making Meaning of Addiction from the Perspective of People in Recovery for Opioid Use Disorder. *Health Communication* 38 (13): 2936–2944. https://doi.org/10.1080/10410236.2022.2128157.

Zelaya, Carla E., James M. Dahlhamer, Jacqueline W. Lucus, and Eric M. Connor. 2020. Chronic Pain and High-Impact Chronic Pain Among US Adults, 2019. *NCHS Data Brief* 390:1–8. https://www.cdc.gov/nchs/products/databriefs/db390.htm.

PART II

Communication and Prevention

CHAPTER 6

Campaign Message Elements for Changing Opioid-Related Behavioral Intent

Braden H. Bagley and Hayden V. Coombs

6.1 Introduction

The opioid crisis remains a formidable public health challenge with deeply impactful social, economic, and healthcare ramifications. In fact, unintentional deaths due to opioid toxicity increased during the pandemic (Gomes et al. 2023, 5). Much of the efforts to bring awareness to the opioid crisis may have been diminished as most people's attention focused on COVID-19. A renewed focus on opioid campaigns can help correct this trend. Effectively addressing the opioid challenge requires strategic communication efforts to change public attitudes and behavioral intent related to opioid use and protection (Voepel-Lewis et al. 2018, 7). This chapter delineates campaign message characteristics that are effective at modifying behavioral intentions and reducing opioid misuse.

Using communication behavioral theories such as the Extended Parallel Process Model (EPPM) and the Health Belief Model (HBM), this chapter emphasizes the necessity of catering to the audience's demographic

B. H. Bagley (✉) • H. V. Coombs
Department of Communication, Southern Utah University, Cedar City, UT, USA
e-mail: bradenbagley@suu.edu; haydencoombs@suu.edu

X. Cao (ed.), *Fighting the Opioid Crisis with Communication*,
https://doi.org/10.1007/978-3-032-31162-7_6

characteristics, behavioral insights, and other psychological factors, such as severity, susceptibility, self-efficacy, and response-efficacy perceptions. Additionally, less-often studied factors such as system-efficacy are considered (Bagley et al. 2022, 5). Recognizing each factor that impacts perceptions of opioids, including stigma and fear, creates a sturdy foundation for campaign messaging (Moore et al. 2020, 808). In order for successful messaging, communicators must effectively transmit useful information that impacts the audience's perception of the threat (opioids) as well as efficacy.

This chapter centers on the strategic crafting of campaign messages that effectively communicate the risks associated with opioid misuse while avoiding the pitfalls of overwhelming individuals with fear and underselling the efficacious elements of the messages. In addition to educating an audience about the dangers of opioid misuse and the efficacious actionable steps they can take to prevent or stop the misuse, the chapter also focuses on encouraging behavior change through supportive and resourceful messaging. While messaging should target all demographics (Schuler et al. 2021, 6), it is also important that messaging is tailored for higher-risk groups, such as men aged 35–44 (National Safety Council 2025). Targeted efforts can help ensure that resources reach those most likely to encounter harm.

This chapter also introduces a list of technical messaging strategies that increase the effectiveness of opioid campaign messaging. These strategies include message framing (i.e., gain/loss), linguistic choices in messaging (i.e., linguistic agency), naming and labeling of victims, social support themes, attention placed on tangible tools and resources, emphasis on negative outcomes such as addiction, family struggles, overdose, stigma, anticipated guilt, financial troubles, and legal repercussions (Bagley and Beckham 2020, 3; Bagley et al. 2022, 5; Cao 2023, 244).

By leveraging insights from communication theory and strategic message design, those tasked with designing opioid campaign messages can significantly influence the fight against the opioid crisis (Richards et al. 2022, 164). As campaigns gain tactical momentum, large-scale changes in behavioral intent can hopefully begin to take place among affected populations. As awareness grows surrounding the negative effects of opioid addiction, the hope is that it follows trends of other addictive substances, such as tobacco smoking, and its misuse will decline with each generation.

6.2 Theoretical Models for Opioid Campaigns

Public health campaigns are most effective when grounded in theory that predicts how people respond to health threats. This chapter highlights two models, including the Extended Parallel Process Model (EPPM) and the Health Belief Model (HBM). The EPPM is particularly valuable when campaigns use fear appeals, a strategy often adopted by health messages about opioids, as it highlights message elements necessary for inducing a danger-control response. In contrast, the HBM offers broader utility for campaigns, not just fear-based messaging. Together, these models provide a strong foundation for designing opioid campaign messaging that is both emotionally resonant and effective.

6.2.1 EPPM

The extended parallel process model (EPPM) is perhaps used more often than any other theory or model in the communication discipline to study fear appeals. The model originated when Kim Witte attempted to clear up the "disappointingly inconsistent, if not contradictory" empirical findings surrounding fear appeal messages (Witte 1992, 329). In the three-plus decades since, the EPPM has been used thousands of times by researchers who similarly want to know how fear can lead people to act. Perhaps one of the finest characteristics of the EPPM is its simplicity in explaining what an effective fear appeal message might look like. The model suggests that four elements should be present for the fear appeal to have its intended effect.

The first message element is threat severity, which communicates that the threat in question (in this case, any threat resulting from opioid use) is dangerous. For example, a message that effectively convinces an individual that opioid use can kill the user should result in a high perception of threat severity. The second element is threat susceptibility, which communicates that the threat in question pertains to the person receiving the message. If the perception of threat susceptibility is high, an individual's response is "this could happen to me."

The third message element is self-efficacy, which communicates that although the threat is real, the ability to overcome it is within an individual's grasp. A person who views or reads an opioid message and then considers themselves capable of overcoming the threat has gained a high perception of self-efficacy. Finally, the fourth element is response-efficacy, which communicates that the recommended response is effective. For instance, if a message about opioids is trying to convince the individual to carry naloxone, and the individual perceives that naloxone is a reliable and effective tool in combating opioid overdose, then they would have a high perception of response-efficacy regarding naloxone.

The EPPM also details the potential outcomes associated with successful and unsuccessful fear appeals. An individual who is exposed to a message that effectively raises the perceptions of both threat (severity and vulnerability) and efficacy (self-efficacy and response-efficacy) is likely to engage in danger control. In this situation, the individual not only understands the threat but is confident in their ability to respond to it. As a result, the individual will likely attempt to control the threat by adhering to the advice offered in the message. If the message adequately raises perceptions of the threat, but fails to raise perceptions of efficacy, then an individual will likely engage in fear control. In this scenario, the individual will attempt to suppress fear via denial ("That won't happen to me"), avoidance ("I don't want to think about it"), or disengagement from the message entirely, leading to an inaction and missed opportunities for prevention. This is not an ideal response. Finally, if the perception of threat is not raised by the message, then there will be no response, regardless of how well the message raises perception of efficacy.

Research into public health campaigns directed toward the opioid crisis has shown that messages developed using the EPPM framework effectively influence a variety of behaviors. These include persuading people to purchase naloxone, increasing youth's intention to talk with parents (Adams et al. 2022, 9–11), and increasing pharmacists' willingness to recommend or dispense over-the-counter naloxone (Thornton et al. 2017, S15). For as long as opioids continue to be a valid threat, fear appeals will have a place in public health campaigns addressing the crisis. With no reason to believe that will change, the EPPM should continue to be used as an effective model for creating and evaluating opioid-related fear appeals.

6.2.2 HBM

Public health campaign messaging combating the opioid crisis extends well beyond fear appeals. Where the EPPM no longer has relevance, the health belief model (HBM) is a useful tool for developing messages that still impact behavioral intent. The model was originally developed to explain preventive health behavior (Rosenstock 1974, 354) and is still used widely today to predict a wide variety of health-related behavior. In addition to being utilized outside of fear appeals, the HBM also separates itself from the EPPM by focusing initially on the inherent demographic and psychological characteristics that an individual brings to the table before a message is even received. This direct acknowledgment of the individual attributes allows the model to better predict behaviors within specific demographic groups, rather than making broad, generalized predictions.

In addition to demographic and psychological characteristics, the health belief model has six variables that predict an individual's likelihood to act on a message, including perceived susceptibility, perceived severity, perceived benefits, perceived barriers, health motivation, and cues to action. Similar to the EPPM, perceived susceptibility and perceived severity are essential variables that measure the individual's respect for the illness, event, or danger that the health message is addressing. Where the HBM really differs from the EPPM is the absence of perceived efficacy as a predicting variable. Instead, the model utilizes perceived benefits and barriers to measure how effective the response being suggested can be at addressing the threat. For instance, a message about naloxone could be unsuccessful if an individual sees minimal benefits of carrying naloxone and sees their inexperience using naloxone as a major barrier to it being effective.

The HBM also considers health motivation as a predicting variable. This variable was introduced to the model to measure the "readiness to be concerned about health matters" (Becker et al. 1977, 40). This variable may be more difficult to influence through typical messaging strategies, as some individuals are simply less concerned with health matters than others. For instance, an individual may find a well-designed opioid public service announcement convincing yet still choose not to act due to low personal motivation or a perceived lack of relevance. However, if the lack of motivation is due to unawareness of occurrences of opioid abuse, it can be addressed in campaigns but might still be difficult to overcome.

Assuming the proper message elements are in place and health motivation is high, cues to action (or calls-to-action) should lead to a high rate of compliance with the message's recommendations. In opioid campaigns, the call-to-action could include a myriad of responses such as carrying naloxone, calling an addiction hotline, telling a friend or family member about one's situation, and properly disposing of old prescription bottles. Regardless of which directions the campaign is directed, an effective theoretical model should always be employed to guide the design of the messaging. Although other models can also be excellent options for preparing campaign messaging, the EPPM and the HBM are perhaps the two models most uniquely tailored to address public health issues such as the opioid crisis.

6.2.3 System-Efficacy

Nearly all models that attempt to explain health behavior use perceived efficacy as a predicting variable, splitting efficacy into self-efficacy and response-efficacy. For example, as explained above, the EPPM uses these two measurements to quantify an individual's overall level of perceived efficacy (Witte 1992). Recently, however, system-efficacy has been introduced and used as an additional measurement that adds to total efficacy. System-efficacy considers the organizations, entities, support network, and other forces at play within the system(s) that an individual is a part of (Bagley et al. 2022, 5). For instance, a mother who trusts a school with her child must also trust a bus driver, teacher, classmates, other parents, a school district, curriculum designers, and many other entities that affect the entire school system. Her perception of how effective that system is at protecting her child plays into her total perception of efficacy, along with self-efficacy and response-efficacy.

Almost any public health campaign can benefit from messaging that heightens an individual's perception of system-efficacy. For example, campaigns that encourage vaccination, whether it be COVID-19, flu, or other vaccines, may benefit from messaging that puts minds at ease about the roles that pharmaceutical companies and the government entities play in the vaccine development and approval process by emphasizing the rigorous clinical trials and review process that lead to the approval of each vaccine (Wentzell and Racila 2021). Similarly, a campaign encouraging people to wear sunscreen could also benefit from messaging that addresses the trustworthiness of companies manufacturing the product and safeness of the ingredients used. In either of these two cases, people consider their trust (or distrust) in the system they belong to when making decisions about their health.

System-efficacy has been found to be a significant predictor of behavioral intent for messages addressing the opioid crisis and, in some cases, more impactful than self-efficacy (Bagley et al. 2022). This could be because protective actions for addressing opioid overdose, such as carrying naloxone, are often measures taken to protect others, not oneself. For instance, if people carry naloxone, they are doing so to help others who overdose. “When a perceived threat is more likely to affect other people in our social circles but not us directly, system-efficacy is a better predictor than self-efficacy” (Bagley et al. 2022, 12). Therefore, models used to inform the creation of opioid-related messages should consider the inclusion of system-efficacy as a variable.

6.3 Messaging Strategies

Theory provides a foundation of understanding how individuals respond to health messages. But the actual crafting of campaign messages requires deliberate strategies. This section introduces specific messaging strategies that take principles from theory and research. These strategies— ranging from framing and language choices, to how stigma is addressed, and consequences are portrayed—help shape how messages are received, interpreted, and acted upon by the audience. If these strategies are adopted by campaign messages, the messages will likely raise awareness and influence behavior in a meaningful way.

6.3.1 Gain/Loss Framing

Framing a message using either the gain-frame or loss-frame technique refers to the way risk is expressed in a message using either positive or negative content in order to persuade someone to adopt a behavior (Cho and Boster 2008, 429). The gain-frame technique highlights what an individual can gain from adhering to the message’s recommendation. For instance, the promise of beautiful white teeth to anyone who commits to flossing and brushing their teeth every day is a gain frame. The loss-frame technique, on the other hand, emphasizes what an individual could lose if they fail to heed the message’s recommendation. Gingivitis, yellow teeth, or missing teeth are some of the outcomes that could be mentioned in a loss-framed tooth brushing and flossing campaign message.

In opioid campaigns, both types of framing can be used. Gain-frame messages can focus on freedom from addiction, clearer focus, more energy, and other benefits from abstaining from painkillers, heroin etc. However, it’s more common to find loss-frame messages in such campaigns, as there is a lot to lose from an opioid addiction. These messages often highlight some of the most significant consequences of opioid addiction, including stigma, family struggles, overdose, guilt, financial troubles, and legal troubles, which are all outlined later in this chapter. A recent study by one of the authors of this chapter found that loss-framed messages were more effective than gain-framed messages at increasing perceptions of threat, which in turn predicted a stronger intention to carry naloxone (Bagley et al. 2022). The finding suggests that emphasizing what could be lost, such as a loved one, may raise perceived severity, making protective actions like carrying naloxone feel more urgent and necessary. Future research may explore whether a loss-frame message is more effective among message recipients who lack the necessary perceived severity of or susceptibility to opioid addiction and abuse.

Loss-framed messages are especially common in campaigns designed to prevent opioid misuse. These messages often highlight the negative consequences of opioid misuse, such as addiction, overdose, fractured relationships, financial ruin, and legal problems. When appropriately communicated, these consequences are often compelling motivators. Loss-framed messaging can be particularly persuasive when paired with high perceived severity and susceptibility, as outlined earlier in the chapter. When individuals believe that severe negative outcomes can happen to them, they are more likely to engage in protective behaviors (Bagley et al. 2022).

However, negative outcomes must be communicated carefully. Overly dramatic or fear-inducing messages can backfire if not balanced by perceived efficacy (Witte and Allen 2000, 606). Messages that rely solely on fear may cause avoidance or denial rather than action. The most effective campaigns pair vivid portrayals of consequences with concrete steps audiences can take to avoid them. In doing so, they maintain urgency while still empowering individuals to act. More specific examples of communicating negative outcomes and specific steps that the audience can take are outlined in the sections below.

6.3.2 Linguistic Assignment of Agency

The concept of linguistic assignment of agency was originally introduced to the health communication literature by McGlone et al. (2013, 741). The premise of this message characteristic is the assignment of the ability to act to either the human or the threat in the message. For instance, a message about COVID-19 that utilizes human-agency would say something like, "You can catch COVID-19 if you go to big group events." The emphasis is placed on "you" the human and the ability of the human to catch the virus. A threat-agency message could say, "COVID-19 will infect people at big group events." The emphasis now being on COVID-19's ability to infect people.

Using threat-agency assignment has been consistently shown to increase perceived severity and behavioral intention (McGlone et al. 2024, 2). This was the case in a study on the opioid epidemic from 2022 which revealed severity to be a significant moderator between agency and behavioral intent when the linguistic agency was assigned to opioids and not to humans (Bagley et al. 2022, 11). The messages used in the study were meant to persuade people to carry Narcan, a naloxone product. The threat-agentic messages used statements like, "Opioid pills and heroin killed over 63,000 victims." The emphasis was clearly placed on the ability of opioid to kill. The human-agentic messages used statements like, "Over 63,000 people died from opioid pills and heroin." The emphasis of the latter messages was clearly placed on an individual's ability to die from opioids. The threat-agentic messages were significantly more impactful, but the effect was conditional on high perceived severity. In other words, the messages only led to increased behavioral intent when individuals already perceived opioid misuse as a serious threat.

6.3.3 Naming and Labeling of Victims

The language used to describe individuals affected by opioid use carries significant weight in shaping public perception, policy, and behavioral intent. Labels such as *addict*, *abuser*, or *junkie* often carry stigma that can reduce a person's identity to their addiction, framing them poorly in the eyes of others, while terms like *victim*, *patient*, or *individual struggling with opioid use* can humanize people and emphasize the nature of the crisis as one less associated with criminal behavior (Goodyear et al. 2018, 2; Ashford et al. 2019, 51). The choice between labeling someone an *abuser* versus a *victim* can influence whether an audience perceives the individual as someone deserving of help or blame.

Research has shown that language has the power to both inflate and deflate stigma surrounding substance use disorders. Kelly and associates (2015, 8) emphasize this point well:

> *Use of the more medically and scientifically accurate 'substance use disorder' terminology is linked to a public health approach that captures the medical malfunction inherent in addiction. Use of this term may decrease stigma and increase help-seeking. In contrast, tough, punitive language, including the*

> *word 'war,' in 'war on drugs,' is intended to send an uncompromising message, 'You use, you lose,' in the hopes of deterring drug involvement.*

Campaigns that employ stigmatizing labels may inadvertently increase misconceptions and reduce the likelihood that others will intervene, support, or advocate for affected individuals (Tsai et al. 2019). Conversely, compassionate, humanizing language has been shown to increase empathy and support for solutions (Kelly and Westerhoff 2010). For example, referring to someone as a *victim of opioid addiction* places emphasis on the systemic factors at play, rather than personal failings.

In opioid campaign messaging, careful attention must be given to naming conventions. A label is not merely a descriptor, but a cue that primes the audience's emotional response (Bagley et al. 2022). By framing individuals as victims, campaign designers can encourage more compassionate behavior from message recipients, which will in turn lead to increases in advocacy and community support. Language is not neutral in the context of opioid messaging but is one of the most powerful tools a campaign designer has available.

6.3.4 Social Support, Tangible Tools, and Resources

Integrating social support themes into opioid misuse prevention campaigns can have a measurable positive impact on their success. Individuals grappling with opioid misuse often experience social isolation, which can hinder recovery efforts (Christie 2021, 652). By highlighting the availability of support networks such as family, friends, healthcare professionals, and community groups, campaigns can mitigate the feeling of isolation and encourage people struggling with addiction to seek assistance.

Effective messaging should not only suggest that support exists but also provide clear guidance on how to find it. Including information about hotlines, addiction recovery services, and social media support groups can be a useful call-to-action employed in campaign messaging. For instance, community-driven responses have been shown to be essential in ensuring the adoption and sustainability of evidence-based practices that can reduce fatal overdoses (El-Bassel et al. 2021, 14).

Moreover, framing social support as a reciprocal process can further enhance campaign impact. Encouraging individuals not only to seek help but also to offer support by learning to administer naloxone and recognize signs of overdose, or engaging with peers in recovery, can foster a sense of shared responsibility (Perreault et al. 2021). Incorporating these elements into opioid prevention campaigns can create a more supportive environment that encourages individuals to seek help and participate actively in their recovery journey.

In addition to the emotional and social support tools mentioned above, opioid campaigns are strengthened by communicating other specific and tangible resources that one can use to protect themselves. While social support messaging emphasizes connection, this approach focuses on actionable solutions such as naloxone kits, drug disposal drop boxes, fentanyl test strips, and safe-use education materials (Fischer et al. 2025). When campaigns point audiences to these tangible resources, they enhance perceived response-efficacy by helping individuals see a clear solution. These short-term calls-to-action can also give struggling victims a sense of victory by allowing them to check a box of accomplishment that comes with following through on an action to help themselves.

This type of messaging is particularly effective when it clearly explains how these tools can be used in a real-life situation. Simply knowing that naloxone exists is not enough, for example. Individuals need to know where to get it, how to use it, and why it matters. Campaigns that offer clear, step-by-step instructions can significantly improve outcomes. For instance, research has shown that people are more likely to carry and administer naloxone when they receive brief, practical training on its use (Green et al. 2008, 6). The presence of tangible resources not only builds individual confidence for those hesitant to intervene but also helps normalize protective behaviors like carrying naloxone, which builds a culture of prevention.

The inclusion of visible tools in campaign messaging can help normalize protective behaviors (Fischer et al. 2025). Just as carrying a first-aid kit or wearing sunscreen is viewed as responsible and proactive, carrying Narcan or using a medication lockbox should be framed as standard actions. Normalization reduces stigma, encourages adoption, and creates a more prevention-minded culture.

6.3.5 *Communicating Consequences of Opioid Misuse*

6.3.5.1 Tailoring Messages to Family Dynamics

Family members play a central, yet often overlooked, role in the public health narrative surrounding opioid misuse. When campaign messages highlight the emotional and relational toll of opioid misuse on family systems, they have the potential to deepen public understanding and encourage broader community support (O'Shay et al. 2023, 103). Research shows that affected family members experience "courtesy stigma," where they are blamed, judged, or socially distanced due to their association with someone who misuses opioids (Alhussain et al. 2019, 9; O'Shay et al. 2023, 90). These stigmas can erode family communication, emotional health, and cohesion, ultimately compromising the very support systems essential for recovery. Campaigns that effectively illuminate these struggles without assigning blame can humanize the crisis and mobilize compassion-driven action.

Effective health communication messaging should also recognize and validate the diverse communication dynamics within families. Kemp et al. (2024, 89) found that families with lower levels of open communication responded better to messages encouraging indirect approaches, such as non-confrontational conversations or leading by example, when addressing a loved one's opioid use. Conversely, high-conversation families were receptive to both direct and indirect messaging. This underscores the importance of tailoring communication strategies to fit each family's cultural dialogue norms. Given that family cohesion has been shown to positively influence both communication and overall well-being, even in the presence of opioid misuse, campaigns should include messages that encourage building strong familial bonds, fostering emotional openness, and accessing resources together (Alhussain et al. 2019, 9; Pasman et al. 2024, 435). Campaigns that portray family struggles in nuanced, stigma-reducing ways do not only foster greater empathy but also inspire community-driven solutions rooted in resilience and care. For example, a campaign might feature a short video of a mother navigating her son's recovery journey. Instead of focusing solely on the son's addiction, the story emphasizes the family's challenges while also showing how they rebuild trust. By highlighting both the pain and the healing process, the campaign avoids blame and instead creates empathy, showing audiences that recovery is a shared, community-supported effort rather than an individual endeavor.

6.3.5.2 Overdose Messaging

Few outcomes of opioid use are as devastating and impactful as an overdose. Campaigns that effectively communicate the realities of overdose, including its rapid onset, unpredictability, and fatal potential, can increase the public's desire to fight the epidemic (Luster 2025). Simply pointing to the statistics surrounding overdose does not maximize the effect that the message can have. Messages should incorporate vivid, real-world scenarios to make the risk feel authentic and personal. When audiences understand (1) how quickly an overdose can occur, (2) how often it happens in everyday environments, and (3) who is overdosing, they're more likely to engage in protective behaviors like carrying naloxone or avoiding opioids altogether.

It's also important that overdose messaging avoids overemphasis on fatality. Instead, focusing on the fact that overdose is preventable, treatable, and survivable with quick intervention helps the audience maintain a sense of control, or self-efficacy. Campaigns should prioritize calls-to-action to accomplish this balancing act. For instance, teaching the audience how to recognize signs of overdose, how to respond effectively, and how to access and use life-saving resources like naloxone are all examples of useful calls-to-action. Using proven campaign methods, like the *Prepare-Plan-Implement* process, can provide structure to accomplish these objectives (Lefebvre et al. 2020, 2). The goal is not just to induce fear of overdosing, but to prepare misusers and their loved ones for potential overdoses.

6.3.5.3 Emotional Barriers

Stigma remains one of the most persistent barriers to opioid recovery and prevention efforts (Tsai et al. 2019). Negative social judgments about individuals who misuse opioids often result in shame, secrecy, and avoidance of treatment. When campaigns fail to address stigma, or worse, reinforce it, they can push individuals further into isolation (Cheetham et al. 2022). Messaging that addresses stigma head on, and promotes healthy discussion around the topic, can help dismantle it at the community level, and diminish its power at the individual level.

Using some of the tactics already discussed in this chapter, like labeling and naming (e.g., "victim" vs. "addict"), framing (gain-frame vs. loss-frame), and linguistic agency (human-agency vs. threat-agency), stigma can be addressed indirectly in campaign messaging. Of course, campaign messaging can address stigma directly as well, by highlighting the roles all individuals play in each other's trauma and mental health outcomes. Using real stories from individuals in recovery can humanize the issue and reduce social distance between those who struggle with opioid misuse and those who don't. *The Truth* (n.d.) campaign accomplished this successfully with a message named *Rebekkah's Story* that publicly displayed the detox experience of an opioid victim named Rebekkah. Her vulnerability and willingness to be the face of opioid detox humanized opioid victims in the minds of those who watched her going through the experience while it was happening. Reducing stigma is essential to overcoming the global battle with opioid misuse. Scientific evidence supports this narrative-based approach. Adams et al. (2022, 8) found that narratives using emotional flow sequences—specifically shifting from threat to efficacy—elicited greater hope and self-efficacy among youth exposed to anti-opioid messaging. Likewise, Cook et al. (2014, 107) demonstrated that interventions at the interpersonal level, such as dyadic storytelling or small-group engagement, can meaningfully reduce stigma and create ripple effects across broader social systems. Moreover, though focused on HIV, Obeagu and Obeagu (2024, 11) emphasized that stigma reduction through real-life storytelling, education, and humanization is a transferable strategy across public health contexts, including substance use. Collectively, this body of research confirms that real-life recovery stories—when strategically implemented—can play a powerful role in reducing stigma and increasing campaign efficacy.

Incorporating scenarios that prompt audiences to reflect on potential emotional consequences of their behavior can also enhance the effectiveness of opioid messages. Anticipated guilt is one of these emotional consequences. Anticipated guilt is the preemptive feeling of remorse for a potential action and can be a powerful motivator for those trying to combat opioid addiction (Cao 2023, 244). When an individual considers the possibility of abusing opioids and predicts the guilt that will follow, they may be more inclined to resist the temptation when it comes. This can be accomplished in campaign messaging by employing narratives from individuals dealing with these temptations. As the character expresses the guilt they feel from their opioid dependence, the audience is invited to imagine themselves in a similar situation. By strategically highlighting anticipated guilt in campaign messaging, we can encourage proactive decision-making and provide confidence to victims that they have the capacity to prevent misuse before it happens. This approach not only informs but also emotionally engages the audience, fostering a deeper personal commitment to avoiding harmful behaviors. Indeed, Cao (2023, 244) found that anticipated guilt aroused by anti-opioid messaging significantly increased the intentions to avoid misusing prescription opioids among young adults. Like anticipated guilt, hope can also be motivational when used in a structured narrative (Adams et al. 2022). Emotional shifts in narrative messaging, particularly from fear to hope, can increase self-efficacy and intention to act. Together, these findings affirm that emotionally driven messages, whether referring to anticipated guilt or hope, can enhance audience engagement and message effectiveness.

6.3.5.4 *Financial and Legal Consequences*

Opioid misuse often carries steep financial consequences for those affected (Warth et al. 2020; Hastert et al. 2023). As addiction deepens, individuals may prioritize drug acquisition over essential expenses, leading to missed housing payments, job loss, and debt accumulation. For many, the long-term economic fallout includes depleted savings, loss of insurance coverage, and a reliance on public resources. These consequences don't just affect the victims, but they ripple out to families and communities, compounding hardship and deepening cycles of poverty. Research shows that when financial hardship becomes overwhelming, individuals are less likely to seek help or maintain treatment—a pattern evident in broader healthcare contexts as well. When campaigns highlight these financial struggles, they add a practical, relatable layer of deterrence to the emotional and physical risks already emphasized.

While much of the research on financial hardship in healthcare settings focuses on systemic barriers to care (Hastert et al. 2023), the principle remains the same: when economic strain becomes overwhelming, individuals are less likely to seek help or maintain treatment. Studies show that stigma, low health literacy, and lack of provider training all contribute to the silence around financial hardship, even when it's a major driver of health behaviors (Warth et al. 2020, 7). Campaigns that clearly connect opioid misuse with tangible financial loss, credit damage, job instability, legal fees, and medical debt can resonate powerfully, especially with financially deprived audiences. Bringing money into the conversation makes it more urgent and real to the audience.

Effective communication about the legal implications of opioid misuse is essential in both medical and public health contexts yet often overlooked in prevention campaigns (Shomaker and Ashburn 2000). Healthcare communication intersects with legal considerations such as informed consent, breach of confidentiality, and defamation (Shomaker and Ashburn 2000, 94). For instance, the use of medical records to document patient histories, including substance use, can expose both the patient and provider to legal vulnerabilities if not handled carefully. Campaigns that aim to raise awareness about opioid use should take these legal dynamics into account by clearly explaining patients' rights, the boundaries of provider confidentiality, and the implications of law enforcement or insurance-related disclosures (Shomaker and Ashburn 2000, 94). Transparency about how legal outcomes, including arrest, litigation, or denial of coverage, can follow certain opioid-related behaviors may help patients and their families make more informed, precautionary decisions.

Moreover, public communication campaigns must navigate the complex terrain of risk communication in ways that ethically balance public safety with individual rights. Bagley and Coombs (2024, 448) highlight that health communication increasingly involves managing sensitive disclosures and legal protections. This includes not only informing patients and the public of the legal risks associated with opioid misuse, such as possession charges or fraud in prescription use, but also ensuring that campaign messaging does not violate privacy laws or stigmatize individuals, potentially opening communicators to defamation claims. For marginalized populations and individuals with limited health literacy, legal messaging must be paired with culturally competent communication (Feinberg et al. 2021, 45). Doing so ensures that vulnerable groups can understand the legal stakes involved while preserving trust in the systems meant to protect them. These approaches underscore the need for opioid campaigns to adopt communication strategies that are not only persuasive and educational, but also legally sound and ethically responsible.

6.4 Conclusion

The opioid crisis remains one of the most pressing public health challenges of the twenty-first century, and the messaging strategies we employ in response can significantly influence both perception and behavior. Campaigns that rely on sound theoretical frameworks, such as the EPPM and HBM, are better equipped to create messages that both educate the public and lead to better decision-making and self-protection. When messages successfully balance fear with efficacy and speak directly to the experiences of victims and loved ones, they are more likely to lead to positive change.

Each element explored in this chapter, whether it's the label we assign to opioid users, the emotional weight of anticipated guilt, or the practical burden of financial loss, plays a distinct role in shaping public understanding and behavioral intent. Health campaigns are not about fear or empty slogans. Instead, the role of campaign designers is to craft messages that are honest, empathetic, and actionable. By carefully designing messages that resonate with the realities of those most affected, communicators have the power to reverse the trends of opioid misuse.

References

Adams, Elizabeth Troutman, Robin L. Nabi, Seth M. Noar, Reina Evans, and Laura Widman. 2022. How Emotional Shifts Affect Youth Perceptions of Opioid Risk and Efficacy: Testing a Know the Truth Campaign Narrative. *Health communication* 37 (14): 1820–1831. https://doi.org/10.1080/10410236.2021.1921349.

Alhussain, Khalid, Drishti Shah, James Douglas Thornton, and Kimberly M. Kelly. 2019. Familial Opioid Misuse and Family Cohesion: Impact on Family Communication and Well-being. *Addictive Disorders & Their Treatment* 18 (4): 194–204. https://doi.org/10.1097/ADT.0000000000000165.

Ashford, Robert David, Austin Brown, and Brenda Curtis. 2019. Expanding Language Choices to Reduce Stigma: A Delphi Study of Positive and Negative Terms in Substance use and Recovery. *Health Education* 119 (1): 51–62. https://doi.org/10.1108/HE-03-2018-0017.

Bagley, Braden H., and Jessica Beckham. 2020. Building Messages for the Opioid Crisis Using the Extended Parallel Process Model. *Qualitative Research Reports in Communication* 22 (1): 47–55. https://doi.org/10.1080/17459435.2020.1836017.

Bagley, Braden H., and Hayden V. Coombs. 2024. Health Communication. In *Encyclopedia of Sports Management,* edited by Paul M. Pedersen. Edward Elgar Publishing. https://doi.org/10.4337/9781035317189.ch262.

Bagley, Braden H., Kathryn Anthony, and Steven Venette. 2022. Framing, Agency, and Optimistic Bias: Message Design Considerations for the Opioid Crisis. *Communication Research and Practice* 8 (4): 347–363. https://doi.org/10.1080/22041451.2022.2143665.

Becker, Marshall H., Don P. Haefner, Stanislav V. Kasl, John P. Kirscht, Lois A. Maiman, and Irwin M. Rosenstock. 1977. Selected Psychosocial Models and Correlates of Individual Health-Related Behaviors. *Medical care* 15 (5): 27–46. https://doi.org/10.1097/00005650-197705001-00005.

Cao, Xiaoxia. 2023. The Impacts of the Reference Focus of Anti-Prescription Opioid Campaigns on Young Americans: The Roles of Anticipated Guilt and Psychological Reactance. *Atlantic Journal of Communication* 31 (4): 312–324. https://doi.org/10.1080/15456870.2022.2081691.

Cheetham, Ali, Louisa Picco, Anthony Barnett, Dan I. Lubman, and Suzanne Nielsen. 2022. The Impact of Stigma on People with Opioid Use Disorder,

Opioid Treatment, and Policy. *Substance Abuse and Rehabilitation* 13 (1): 1–12. https://doi.org/10.2147/SAR.S304566.
Cho, Hyunyi, and Franklin J. Boster. 2008. Effects of Gain Versus Loss Frame Antidrug Ads on Adolescents. *Journal of Communication* 58 (3): 428–446. https://doi.org/10.1111/j.1460-2466.2008.00393.x.
Christie, Nina C. 2021. The Role of Social Isolation in Opioid Addiction. *Social Cognitive and Affective Neuroscience* 16 (7): 645–656. https://doi.org/10.1093/scan/nsab029.
Cook, Judith E., Valerie Purdie-Vaughns, Ilan H. Meyer, and Jennifer T. Busch. 2014. Intervening Within and Across Levels: A Multilevel Approach to Stigma and Public Health. *Social Science & Medicine* 103:101–109. https://doi.org/10.1016/j.socscimed.2013.09.023.
El-Bassel, Nabila, Louisa Gilbert, Tim Hunt, et al. 2021. Using Community Engagement to Implement Evidence-Based Practices for Opioid Use Disorder: A Data-Driven Paradigm & Systems Science Approach. *Drug and Alcohol Dependence* 222 (1): 1–22. https://doi.org/10.1016/j.drugalcdep.2021.108675.
Feinberg, Iris Z., Ashli Owen-Smith, Mary Helen O'Connor, Michelle M. Ogrodnick, Richard Rothenberg, and Michael P. Eriksen. 2021. Strengthening Culturally Competent Health Communication. *Health security* 19 (S1): S41–S49. https://doi.org/10.1089/hs.2021.0048.
Fischer, Leah S., Alice Asher, Renee Stein, et al. 2025. Effectiveness of Naloxone Distribution in Community Settings to Reduce Opioid Overdose Deaths among People who use Drugs: A systematic Review and Meta-Analysis. *BMC Public Health* 25 (1): 1135. https://doi.org/10.1186/s12889-025-22210-8.
Gomes, Tara, Shaleesa Ledlie, and Mina Tadrous. 2023. Trends in Opioid Toxicity-related Deaths in the US Before and After the Start of the COVID-19 Pandemic, 2011-2021. *JAMA Network Open* 6 (7): 1–7. https://doi.org/10.1001/jamanetworkopen.2023.22303.
Goodyear, Kimberly, Carolina L. Haass-Koffler, and David Chavanne. 2018. Opioid Use and Stigma: The Role of Gender, Language and Precipitating Events. *Drug and Alcohol Dependence* 185 (1): 339–346. https://doi.org/10.1016/j.drugalcdep.2017.12.037.
Green, Traci C., Robert Heimer, and Lauretta E. Grau. 2008. Distinguishing Signs of Opioid Overdose and Indication for Naloxone: An Evaluation of Six Overdose Training and Naloxone Distribution Programs in the United States. *Addiction* 103 (6): 979–989. https://doi.org/10.1111/j.1360-0443.2008.02182.x.
Hastert, Theresa A., Mrudula Nair, and Susan Eggly. 2023. Providers' Communication-Related Concerns in Helping Patients Address the Financial Impact of Cancer. *Patient Education and Counseling* 114 (1): 107860. https://doi.org/10.1016/j.pec.2023.107860.
Kelly, John F., and Cassandra M. Westerhoff. 2010. Does it Matter How We Refer to Individuals with Substance-Related Conditions? A Randomized Study of

Two Commonly Used Terms. *International Journal of Drug Policy* 21 (3): 202–207. https://doi.org/10.1016/j.drugpo.2009.10.010.

Kelly, John F., Sarah E. Wakeman, and Richard Saitz. 2015. Stop Talking 'Dirty': Clinicians, Language, and Quality of Care for the Leading Cause of Preventable Death in the United States. *The American journal of medicine* 128 (1): 8–9. https://doi.org/10.1016/j.amjmed.2014.07.043.

Kemp, Deena, Mike Mackert, Siyan Li, et al. 2024. Talking about Prescription Opioid Misuse: The Effect of Family Communication Patterns and Messages Advocating Direct and Indirect Communication. *Health Communication* 39 (1): 83–95. https://doi.org/10.1080/10410236.2022.2159136.

Lefebvre, R. Craig, Redonna K. Chandler, Donald W. Helme, et al. 2020. Health Communication Campaigns to Drive Demand for Evidence-Based Practices and Reduce Stigma in the HEALing Communities Study. *Drug and Alcohol Dependence* 217 (1): 108338. https://doi.org/10.1016/j.drugalcdep.2020.108338.

Luster, Jamie. 2025. *Evidence-Based Strategies and Communication Campaigns Help Communities Reduce Overdose Deaths and Addiction Stigma*. The Ohio State University College of Medicine. https://medicine.osu.edu/news/evidence-based-strategies-and-communication-campaigns-help-communities-reduce-overdose-deaths-and-addiction-stigma.

McGlone, Matthew S., Robert A. Bell, Sarah T. Zaitchik, and I. I. I. Joseph McGlynn. 2013. Don't Let the Flu Catch You: Agency Assignment in Printed Educational Materials about the H1N1 Influenza Virus. *Journal of Health Communication* 18 (6): 740–756. https://doi.org/10.1080/10810730.2012.727950.

McGlone, Matthew S., Keri K. Stephens, Mian Jia, Carolyn Montagnolo, and Xu. Yifan. 2024. Multiple Messaging Strategies for Increasing HPV Vaccination Intentions Among English-and Spanish-Speaking Parents in the United States and Mexico. *Vaccines* 12 (6): 650. https://doi.org/10.3390/vaccines12060650.

Moore, Matthew D., Shabana Ali, Danielle Burnich-Line, Whitney Gonzales, and Michael V. Stanton. 2020. Stigma, Opioids, and Public Health Messaging: The Need to Disentangle Behavior from Identity. *American Journal of Public Health* 110 (6): 807–810. https://doi.org/10.2105/AJPH.2020.305628.

National Safety Council. 2025. *Drug Overdoses*. https://injuryfacts.nsc.org/home-and-community/safety-topics/drugoverdoses/#:~:text=The%2035%2D%20to%2044%2Dyear,and%20older%20is%20growing%20rapidly.

O'Shay, Sydney, Emily Pasman, Danielle L. Hicks, Suzanne Brown, Elizabeth Aguis, and Stella M. Resko. 2023. Affected Family Members' Communicative Management of Opioid Misuse Stigma: Applying and Rethinking the Stigma Management Communication Typology. *Journal of Family Communication* 23 (2): 89–106. https://doi.org/10.1080/15267431.2023.2186882.

Obeagu, Elijah I., and Godwin U. Obeagu. 2024. Unmasking the Truth: Addressing Stigma in the Fight Against HIV. *Elite Journal of Public Health* 2 (1): 8–22. https://epjournals.com/journals/EJPH.

Pasman, Emily, Sydney O'Shay, Danielle Hicks, Stella M. Resko, Elizabeth Agius, and Suzanne Brown. 2024. Stigma Communication Surrounding Nonmedical Opioid Use Among Affected Family Members. *Health Communication* 39 (3): 429–438. https://doi.org/10.1080/10410236.2023.2167588.

Perreault, Michel, Marie-Anne Ferlatte, Ana Carolina Artunduaga, Chantale Perron, Carley Marshall, and Diana Milton. 2021. Impact of Participation in a Peer-Led Overdose Program for People Who Use Drugs. *Drugs: Education, Prevention and Policy* 30 (3): 259–268. https://doi.org/10.1080/09687637.2022.2030302.

Richards, Georgia C., Sibtain Anwar, and Jane Quinlan. 2022. Averting a UK Opioid Crisis: Getting the Public Health Messages 'Right'. *Journal of the Royal Society of Medicine* 115 (5): 161–164. https://doi.org/10.1177/01410768221089015.

Rosenstock, Irwin M. 1974. The Health Belief Model and Preventive Health Behavior. *Health Education Monographs* 2 (4): 354–386. https://doi.org/10.1177/109019817400200405.

Schuler, Megan S., Terry L. Schell, and Eunice C. Wong. 2021. Racial/ethnic Differences in Prescription Opioid Misuse and Heroin Use Among a National Sample. *Drug and Alcohol Dependence* 221 (1): 108588. https://doi.org/10.1016/j.drugalcdep.2021.108588.

Shomaker, Samuel T., and Michael A. Ashburn. 2000. The Legal Implications of Healthcare communications: What Every Pain Physician Needs to Know. *Pain Medicine* 1 (1): 89–96. https://doi.org/10.1046/j.1526-4637.2000.99108.x.

The Truth. (n.d.). Rebekkah's Story. https://www.thetruth.com/video/rebekkah-s-story.

Thornton, Douglas J., Elizabeth Lyvers, Virginia Ginger Scott, and Nilanjana Dwibedi. 2017. Pharmacists' Readiness to Provide Naloxone in Community Pharmacies in West Virginia. *Journal of the American Pharmacists Association* 57 (2): S12–S18. https://doi.org/10.1016/j.japh.2016.12.070.

Tsai, Alexander C., Mathew V. Kiang, Michael L. Barnett, et al. 2019. Stigma as a Fundamental Hindrance to the United States Opioid Overdose Crisis Response. *PloS Med* 16 (11): e1002969. https://doi.org/10.1371/journal.pmed.1002969.

Voepel-Lewis, Terri, Brian J. Zikmund Fisher, Carol J. Boyd, et al. 2018. Effects of a Scenario-tailored Opioid Messaging Program on Parents' Risk Perceptions and Opioid Decision Making. *The Clinical Journal of Pain* 34 (6): 497–504. https://doi.org/10.1097/AJP.0000000000000570.

Warth, Jacqueline, Marie-Therese Puth, Ulrike Zier, et al. 2020. Patient-Physician Communication about Financial Problems: A Cross-Sectional Study Among

Over-Indebted Individuals. *PLOS ONE* 15 (5): e0232716. https://doi.org/10.1371/journal.pone.0232716.
Wentzell, Emily, and Ana-Monica Racila. 2021. The Social Experience of Participation in a COVID-19 Vaccine Trial: Subjects' Motivation, Others' Concerns, and Insights for Vaccine Promotion. *Vaccine* 39 (17): 2445–2451. https://doi.org/10.1016/j.vaccine.2021.03.036.
Witte, Kim. 1992. Putting the Fear Back into Fear Appeals: The Extended Parallel Process Model. *Communications Monographs* 59 (4): 329–349. https://doi.org/10.1080/03637759209376276.
Witte, Kim, and Mike Allen. 2000. A Meta-Analysis of Fear Appeals: Implications for Effective Public Health Campaigns. *Health Education & Behavior* 27 (5): 591–615. https://doi.org/10.1177/109019810002700506.

CHAPTER 7

The Immediate and Delayed Impacts of the Reference Focus of Anti-prescription Opioid Risk Narratives: The Mediating Roles of Fear and Anticipated Guilt

Xiaoxia Cao

7.1 Introduction

The American opioid crisis leads to over 220 deaths per day (National Center for Health Statistics 2024) and has cost Americans over $1 trillion every year since 2017 (Beyer 2022). The demographic group that is most negatively affected by the crisis is young Americans (National Safety Council 2022) because of their tendency to engage in risky behaviors (Levy 2019, 3). Even though the crisis is the product of addiction to not only prescription opioids but also heroin and synthetic opioids (e.g., fentanyl), it began with misusing prescription opioids (National Institute on Drug Abuse 2022). For example, 80% of those who use heroin became opioid dependent by misusing prescription opioids first. Hence, one way to combat the opioid crisis is to alert people (especially young people) to the dangers of prescription opioids and discourage them from misusing the drugs via public health campaigns.

X. Cao (✉)
University of Wisconsin-Milwaukee, Milwaukee, WI, USA
e-mail: xcao@uwm.edu

X. Cao (ed.), *Fighting the Opioid Crisis with Communication*, https://doi.org/10.1007/978-3-032-31162-7_7

However, the U.S. government has a long list of failed anti-drug campaigns, especially those targeting young people (Frakt and Humphreys 2017). After reviewing decades of anti-drug campaigns, some scholars have concluded that many of these campaigns were ineffective or even counterproductive (Allara et al. 2015). Thus, it is important to explore how to increase the persuasiveness of anti-prescription opioid campaigns.

Given that the opioid crisis affects not only people with opioid use disorder (OUD) but also those close to them (e.g., their family; Brundage and Levine 2019), some notable anti-prescription opioid campaigns have employed narratives with different reference foci to warn the public of the dangers of (mis)using prescription opioids (e.g., the Rx Awareness campaign by the U.S. Centers for Disease Control and Prevention [CDC] 2021). Narrative is "a representation of connected events and characters that has an identifiable structure, is bounded in space and time, and contains implicit or explicit messages about the topic being addressed" (Kreuter et al. 2007, 22). It often takes on the forms of anecdotes, testimonials, and other stories in health messages (Shen et al. 2015, 105). Narratives that describe risks and/or negative consequences associated with a risky or unhealthy behavior are called risk narratives (Kim and Lee 2018, 2422). The reference focus of health messages is determined by whom a behavior affects, as highlighted in the messages (Cao 2023, 313). Self-focused messages emphasize the impact of one's behavior on oneself (e.g., the death of a person due to OUD); other-focused messages highlight the impact of one's behavior on others who do not engage in the behavior (e.g., the impact of second-hand smoke on nonsmokers); and self-other-focused messages emphasize the impacts of one's behavior on oneself and those who do not engage in the behavior (e.g., the distress experienced by the family members of those who died of opioid overdose).

Thus far, no studies have explored the influence of the reference focus of risk narratives on the persuasiveness of anti-prescription opioid campaigns. Most research into the influence of reference focus has used non-narrative messages and focused on the cognitive explanations for its immediate impact (e.g., psychological reactance, Gardner and Leshner 2016; message elaboration, Hong and Hashimoto 2023; processing fluency and perceived susceptibility, Huang and Li 2023; and message involvement, Li and Rifon 2017; but also see Cao 2023). To improve our understanding of the impacts of the reference focus of risk narratives, this study explores the immediate and delayed attitudinal and behavioral impacts of self-focused versus self-other-focused anti-prescription opioid risk narratives because OUD cannot affect those close to people with the disorder without first negatively affecting the people with the disorder. For example, a mother cannot lose her son to an opioid overdose without her son dying of the overdose first. Thus, anti-prescription opioid messages that recount the negative impacts of OUD on people close to those with OUD often bring attention to the impacts of OUD on not only people close to individuals with the disorder but also those with the disorder (i.e., having a self-other-focus; Cao 2023, 319). Besides investigating the immediate and delayed attitudinal and behavioral impacts of self-focused versus self-other-focused anti-prescription opioid risk narratives, this study also examines the mediating roles of fear and anticipated guilt because risk information can arouse fear (Witte 1992, 331), and imagining oneself having OUD (and hurting others as a result) can arouse anticipated guilt (O'Keefe 2002, 330; Cao 2024, 246). Appealing to fear or anticipated guilt often leads to desired attitudinal and behavioral changes (Witte and Allen 2000; O'Keefe 2002).

This study makes multiple contributions. First, it furthers our understanding of the impacts of the reference focus of risk narratives by being the first to explore the immediate and delayed attitudinal and behavioral impacts of self-focused versus self-other-focused risk narratives. Second, this study is the first to investigate the roles of emotions in explaining the immediate and delayed influence of the reference focus of risk narratives. Third, it answers the call for exploring the influence of multiple emotions aroused simultaneously by persuasive appeals (Carcioppolo et al. 2017, 454) via investigating the roles of fear and anticipated guilt in explaining the impacts of the reference focus of risk narratives. Fourth, by investigating the immediate and delayed attitudinal and behavioral impacts of the reference focus of anti-prescription opioid risk narratives, this study sheds light on strategies that may be used to design effective anti-prescription opioid messages.

7.2 Narrative and Persuasion

Narratives are effective tools for promoting health-related attitudinal and behavioral changes (Shen et al. 2015). Rather than presenting arguments for readers to judge, narratives invite readers to immerse themselves in the real or plausible life experiences of real people or characters that are often difficult to disagree with or dispute. Narrative involvement can exert both cognitive and affective influences on message recipients (Green and Brock

2000). Specifically, such involvement reduces the reader's ability to critically examine messages conveyed by stories. As a result, narratives can overcome various forms of resistance to persuasion (e.g., psychological reactance, counterarguing and perceived invulnerability) and produce message-consistent attitudinal and behavioral changes (Gardner and Leshner 2016; Moyer-Guse and Nabi 2010; Ratcliff and Sun 2020). Moreover, narrative involvement can arouse various emotions among readers that in turn may influence their attitudes and behaviors (Banerjee and Greene 2012; Meadows 2020). There is also evidence that presenting narratives in an overtly (vs. covertly) persuasive context or adding explicit appeals to the end of narratives does not inhibit narrative persuasion (Graaf et al. 2016, 96; Staunton et al. 2022, 617). However, there are significant variations in impacts across narratives with different features (Chen and Bell 2022) and promoting various behaviors (e.g., prevention, detection, or cessation behaviors; Graaf et al. 2016, 91).

7.3 Reference Focus, Risk Narratives, and Persuasion

Current research into the reference focus of persuasive messages has suggested that its impact varies depending upon other message features (e.g., types of appeals, Block 2005; message frames, Loroz 2007; Wong et al. 2015). Two message features that are most relevant to the present study are message frames and narratives given that this study explores the immediate and delayed impacts of the reference focus of anti-prescription opioid risk narratives that are inherently loss framed (i.e., emphasizing the negative consequences of incompliance).

Thus far, no studies have directly tested the influence of the reference focus of risk narratives—determined by who is negatively affected by a risky or unhealthy behavior, as highlighted by the narratives (Cao 2023, 313). Research into the impact of the reference focus of loss-framed non-narrative appeals has shown mixed findings. Some studies have found that when paired with loss frames self-focused (or self-other-focused) appeals are more effective than self-other-focused (or other-focused) appeals in promoting recycling behavior, prevention of sexually transmitted diseases (Loroz 2007), and bystander intervention (Li and Rifon 2017). In explaining the observed persuasive advantage of loss-framed self-focused messages, some scholars contend that self-focused messages help message recipients link the messages to themselves, which increases perceived personal relevance of the messages and message involvement (Loroz 2007, 1016; Li and Rifon 2017, 226; Huang and Li 2023, 389). The increased involvement then leads to persuasion by increasing message elaboration and reducing perceived invulnerability to the negative consequences.

Other studies exploring the influence of the reference focus of non-narrative appeals have found that self-focused loss-framed messages are less effective than their other-focused counterparts (Gardner and Leshner 2016; Cao 2023; Hong and Hashimoto 2023) because the former make message recipients feel threatened (Staunton et al. 2022, 617). Indeed, research has shown that self-focused (vs. other-focused) loss-framed non-narrative messages are considered a threat to personal freedom, elicit counterarguing, and lead to psychological reactance (Gardner and Leshner 2016; Cao 2023). Still others found that the reference focus of non-narrative messages has little impact on reactions to the messages (Ma and Miller 2021).

Even though there is no consensus on how the reference focus of loss-framed non-narrative messages may influence the persuasiveness of such messages and no studies have explored the influence of the reference focus of risk narratives, there are reasons to believe that self-focused risk narratives may be more persuasive than self-other-focused risk narratives. As aforementioned, self-focused loss-framed non-narrative messages sometimes backfire because they induce counterarguing and psychological reactance among message receivers (Gardner and Leshner 2016; Cao 2023). However, this should not happen to self-focused risk narratives because by engaging message recipients in the storyline, such narratives can overcome various forms of resistance to persuasion, including counterarguing, psychological reactance, and perceived invulnerability (Moyer-Guse and Nabi 2010; Ratcliff and Sun 2020).

Moreover, the construal level theory of psychological distance (CLT) suggests that self-focused risk narratives should be more persuasive than self-other-focused risk narratives (Trope and Liberman 2010). According to CLT, individuals can mentally construe the same information, event, or object at different levels, depending upon its perceived psychological distance. When the information, event, or object is perceived to be psychologically close—that is, about the self, here and now—it is represented in a more concrete manner (i.e., at low construal level). As the perceived psychological distance of the information, event, or object increases—that is, about others or moving further away in time or physical distance—it is increasingly represented in a more abstract manner (e.g., at high-level construal). Consequently, risks perceived to be psychologically close as opposed to distant should be represented in a more concrete and vivid manner. The vivid and concrete representation in turn increases perceived seriousness of the risks and compliance (Chandran and Menon 2004). Indeed, research has shown that psychological distance-related factors (e.g., temporal and spatial distance) can be used to manipulate the concreteness of risk communication and, therefore, influence risk perception and behavioral intentions (Chandran and Menon 2004; Yang and McAllister 2020). Given that risks for the self are perceived to be psychologically closer than those involving others, the risk information in self-focused risk narratives should be represented in a more concrete and vivid manner than that in self-other-focused risk narratives as the latter is likely construed in mixed concrete and abstract terms. Consequently, self-focused risk narratives should be more likely than self-other-focused risk narratives to increase risk perceptions and induce desired attitudinal and behavioral changes. For this reason, I propose the following hypotheses:

H1: Exposure to self-focused versus self-other-focused anti-prescription opioid risk narratives will increase (a) negative attitudes toward prescription opioids and (b) intentions to avoid (mis)using the drugs immediately after the exposure.

Given that it is unclear how long the predicted attitudinal and behavioral impacts of the reference focus will last, I ask the following questions:

RQ1: Will the predicted (a) attitudinal and (b) behavioral impacts of exposure to self-focused versus self-other-focused anti-prescription opioid risk narratives still be observed after a period of time (e.g., more than ten days after the exposure)?

7.3.1 The Mediating Roles of Emotions

The role of emotions in explaining the influence of the reference focus of health messages has been understudied (but see Gardner and Leshner 2016; Cao 2023), even though emotions often serve as motivators for changes and can predict attitudes and behaviors over and above cognitive factors (Richard et al. 1996, 125). Emotions are particularly relevant to the present study because narratives are found to influence attitudes and behaviors via arousing various emotions (Banerjee and Greene 2012; Meadows 2020). Thus, this study examines the mediating roles of two emotions—fear and anticipated guilt—that are likely aroused by anti-prescription opioid risk narratives (as elaborated below). Appealing to fear or anticipated guilt often leads to desired attitudinal and behavioral changes (Witte and Allen 2000; O'Keefe 2002).

7.3.2 *The Mediating Role of Fear*

Fear is an emotion experienced when individuals become aware of imminent threat or danger (Witte 1992, 351). It motivates responses that reduce the threat or danger and eliminate the feeling of fear. Meta-analyses have shown that fear aroused by persuasive messages is positively associated with persuasion (White and Albarracin 2018; Witte and Allen 2000). Designers of health messages often appeal to fear by emphasizing the potential danger and harm that will befall message receivers if they do not comply with the recommendations (Tannenbaum et al. 2015, 1179). Thus, anti-prescription opioid risk narratives that highlight the negative consequences of misusing prescription opioids should arouse fear. Such narratives should arouse more fear when they focus on the negative impacts of the misuse on the self (i.e., self-focused) than when they emphasize the negative impacts on the self and others (i.e., self-other-focused). This is because the danger or harm to the self is perceived to be psychologically closer than the danger or harm to others (Trope and Liberman 2010). Consequently, self-focused danger or harm is represented in a more concrete manner than danger or harm involving both the self and others, as the latter is likely construed in mixed concrete and abstract terms. The more concrete representation then makes the danger or harm to the self appear more severe and arouses more fear (Chandran and Menon 2004; Yang and McAllister 2020). Given that fear is a positive predictor of persuasion (White and Albarracin 2018; Witte and Allen 2000), I make the following predictions:

H2: Exposure to self-focused versus self-other-focused anti-prescription opioid risk narratives should arouse more fear immediately after the exposure.

H3: The predicted immediate positive (a) attitudinal and (b) behavioral impacts of exposure to self-focused versus self-other-focused anti-prescription opioid risk narratives should be (partly) explained by the increased fear.

It is unclear whether fear aroused immediately after exposure to the risk narratives will explain the delayed attitudinal and behavioral impacts of the reference focus of such narratives, if the delay impacts are observed. Thus, I ask the following questions:

RQ2: To the extent that the reference focus (self vs. self-other) of anti-prescription opioid risk narratives has delayed (a) attitudinal and (b) behavioral impacts, will the impacts be (partly) explained by increased fear immediately after exposure to the narratives?

7.3.3 The Mediating Role of Anticipated Guilt

Guilt is a negative emotional state experienced when individuals realize that they have violated personal, moral, and/or societal standards that they want to uphold (Carcioppolo et al. 2017, 438). Thus, people likely feel guilty when they have acted in ways inconsistent with their perception of proper conduct (e.g., failing to maintain an exercise plan or hurting others; O'Keefe 2002, 329). Feeling guilty can lead to desired attitudinal and behavioral changes because it motivates individuals to make amends and engage in behaviors that reduce such feeling (Turner 2017, 4).

Anticipated guilt is aroused when people imagine or anticipate their violation of personal, societal, and/or moral standards (Lindsey 2005, 455; Carcioppolo et al. 2017, 438). Health messages appealing to anticipated guilt are effective because anticipated guilt is elicited by imagined or potential future violations of one's perception of proper conduct that can still be avoided (Cao 2024, 246). People are motivated to engage in guilt-reducing behaviors when they believe that doing so can avoid feeling guilty. Consistent with this reasoning, research has shown that individuals' anticipation of feeling guilty, if they engage in risky behaviors, is associated with avoidance of such behaviors (Birkimer et al. 1993, 691; O'Keefe 2002, 334). Moreover, anticipated guilt is found to predict negative attitudes toward prescription opioids and intentions to avoid (mis)using the drugs (Cao 2023, 2024).

OUD is believed by many to be the result of moral failure, even though it can be attributed to multiple factors (Frank and Nagel 2017). Becoming opioid dependent and/or hurting others as a result are arguably against many people's personal and moral standards. Hence, imagining oneself misusing prescription opioids, becoming opioid dependent, and suffering as a result should arouse anticipated guilt and so should imagining harms to others caused by one's OUD. However, self-focused anti-prescription opioid risk narratives should elicit greater anticipated guilt than their self-other-focused counterparts because guilt is found to be aroused in response to concrete representation of specific misconduct (Han et al. 2014, 1049). Given that harm or danger to the self is perceived to be psychologically closer than that involving both the self and others and is construed in a more concrete manner, as suggested by CLT (Trope and Liberman 2010), self-focused (vs. self-other-focused) anti-prescription opioid risk narratives should arouse more anticipated guilt, a positive predictor of negative attitudes toward prescription opioids and intentions to avoid misusing the drugs (Cao 2023, 2024). With all these in mind, I propose the following hypotheses:

H4: Exposure to self-focused versus self-other-focused anti-prescription opioid risk narratives should arouse more anticipated guilt immediately after the exposure.
H5: The predicted immediate positive (a) attitudinal and (b) behavioral impacts of exposure to self-focused versus self-other-focused anti-prescription opioid risk narratives should be (partly) explained by the increased anticipated guilt.

Although guilt appeals in marketing are found to elicit delayed compliance (Antonetti et al. 2018), no studies have explored the delayed impacts of anticipated guilt appeals in the context of health communication. Thus, it is unclear whether anticipated guilt aroused immediately after exposure to the self-focused (vs. self-other-focused) risk narratives will explain the delayed attitudinal and behavioral impacts of the reference focus of such narratives, if the delay impacts are observed. For this reason, I ask the following questions:

RQ3: To the extent that the reference focus (self vs. self-other) of anti-prescription opioid risk narratives has delayed (a) attitudinal and (b) behavioral impacts, will the impacts be (partly) explained by increased anticipated guilt immediately after exposure to the narratives?

7.4 Method

A two-stage randomized online experiment, approved by the Institutional Review Board, was conducted among a convenience sample of college students. The study had a 2 (reference focus: self vs. self-other) X 2 (delay of assessment: short vs. long) mixed design, with the first factor as a between-subjects factor and the second a within-subjects factor. Each study participant read one of four anti-prescription opioid messages. Half of them included a self-focused risk narrative and the other half a self-other-focused risk narrative.

7.4.1 Material

All messages had the same layout. Each included a black-and-white image of hands pouring pills out of a prescription bottle on the left side along with a CDC logo in the lower left corner. On the right side was a story titled "Rx Awareness: [a person's first name]'s story," which described how a person (and the family members of the person) was negatively affected by the person's OUD developed via misusing prescription opioids. Under the story was the campaign message (adopted from the CDC's Rx Awareness campaign 2021), "prescription opioids can be addictive and dangerous. It only takes a little to lose a lot."

The stories used in this study were written based upon real stories of people who were negatively impacted by OUD and obtained from public health campaigns (e.g., Rx Awareness, CDC 2021) and online platforms where people share stories about OUD (e.g., Heroin & Opioid Addiction, in Your Own Words, Public Broadcasting Service 2022). Two stories—each having a self-focused and a self-other-focused version—that varied in the character's gender and the risks highlighted were created to mimic the risk narratives used by real health campaigns, resulting in four messages. Using narratives that varied in the character's gender and risks highlighted enabled me to explore whether the predicted attitudinal and behavioral impacts of the reference focus of risk narratives could extend to stories about different characters and highlighting different risks.

Following the practice of real anti-prescription opioid campaigns (e.g., Rx Awareness; CDC 2021), all stories were presented as testimonials. In the self-focused version, an individual with OUD recounted how s/he became opioid dependent via misusing prescription opioids and how OUD affected his or her life. Participants were told that the person became homeless or died of an overdose. Given that self-other-focused stories concern the experiences of more than one person, the stories could be presented as testimonials from a person with OUD or a family member of such a person. However, it is impossible for individuals with OUD to know how certain consequences of their OUD (e.g., their death) affect their family. Thus, the self-other-focused version of the stories used in this study was told by the mother of a person with OUD (whose story was told in the self-focused version). The mother recounted how her child became opioid dependent and how the dependency affected the child (i.e., becoming homeless or dying of an overdose) and the family (see the appendix for the stories used in the study).

7.4.2 Study Participants and Procedure

Students from entry-level communication courses at two public universities were recruited via email to participate in this study in exchange for extra credit. A total of 77 students participated in the first stage of the study; 53 of them also completed the second stage with a retention rate of 69%. Participants of the first stage had a mean age of 20.38 ($SD = 1.31$); 86% were female; and 70% were white; those of the second stage had a mean age of 20.48 ($SD = 1.13$); 83% were female; and 81% were white.

After accessing the first stage of the study via a link included in the recruitment email and giving informed consent, participants answered questions on their demographics (age, race, and gender), exposure to anti-prescription opioid messages via various media, and experience of misusing prescription opioids before being randomly assigned to read one of the four messages. After reading the message, they completed questions on manipulation check, fear, anticipated guilt, attitudes toward prescription opioids (T1 attitudes), and intentions to avoid (mis)using prescription opioids (T1 intentions). Those who completed the first stage of the study received a link to the second stage of the study ten days after the first stage was closed. During the second stage, they again answered questions about attitudes (T2 attitudes) and behavioral intentions (T2 intentions). The same attitude and behavioral-intention questions were asked at both stages of the study and each stage was open for ten days. The average time lag between the completion of the two stages of the study was 17.32 days ($SD = 3.59$).

7.4.3 Measures

Outcome Variables: Attitudes toward prescription opioids were measured by two items rated on a seven-point agreement scale including, "My attitude toward using prescription opioids is negative," and, "I have an unfavorable view toward using prescription opioids" (1 = strongly disagree; 7 = strongly agree; Cao 2023, 317). Thus, higher scores indicated stronger negative attitudes. An attitude index was created by averaging the ratings on the two items (T1, $M = 5.38$; $SD = 1.37$; $r = 0.73$; T2, $M = 4.90$; $SD = 1.62$; $r = 0.86$). The same method was used to create indices for other variables.

Intentions to avoid (mis)using prescription opioids were measured by three items that gauged the likelihood that participants would engage in three behaviors such as "avoiding misusing prescription opioids at all costs" (1 = very unlikely; 7 = very likely; T1, $M = 5.86$; $SD = 1.22$; $\alpha = 0.70$; T2, $M = 5.72$; $SD = 1.36$; $\alpha = 0.90$; Cao 2023, 317).

Mediators: Fear was measured by asking participants to what extent they felt fearful, scared, or afraid when reading the message (1= not at all; 7 = extremely; $M = 3.11$; $SD = 1.83$; $\alpha = 0.97$; Banerjee and Greene 2012, 571).

Anticipated guilt was assessed by asking participants to what extent they would feel guilty, sorry, regretful, or bad if they started to use (or continued using) prescription opioids from then on ($M = 4.59$; $SD = 2.23$; $\alpha = 0.97$; Cao 2023, 317).

Control Variables: Participants' gender, their prior exposure to anti-prescription opioid messages, and their experience of misusing prescription opioids were included in all analyses as control variables. Participant's gender (male =1; female = 0) was controlled because compared to men, women are more responsive to narratives (Green and Brock 2000) and to fear appeals (Tannenbaum et al. 2015). Prior exposure to anti-prescription opioid campaigns was also controlled because it can influence reactions to persuasive messages on a similar topic (Bigman et al. 2016). The exposure was measured by asking how often participants saw anti-prescription opioid campaigns on various media (1 = never; 4 = often; Oh et al. 2015, 22; $M = 2.05$; $SD = 0.66$; $\alpha = 0.86$). Given that past behavior is a strong positive predictor of future behavior (Fishbein and Ajzen 2009), this study also asked participants how often (1 = never; 4 = often) they had misused prescription opioids (e.g., taking prescription opioids without a prescription) in the past 12 months ($M = 1.06$; $SD = 0.30$; $\alpha = 0.95$; Xu and Cao 2020, 1410; see Table 7.1 for correlations among variables in the analyses).

Manipulation Check: Participants were asked to rate on a seven-point agreement scale two statements including, "The story you just read highlighted the negative impacts of misusing prescription opioids on those who misused them" ($M = 5.49$; $SD = 1.46$) and "on the family members of those who misused them" ($M = 5.04$; $SD = 1.72$).

Table 7.1 Correlations between variables

Variables	*V1*	*V2*	*V3*	*V4*	*V5*	*V6*	*V7*	*V8*	*V9*	*V10*
Independent variable										
1. Reference focus (self vs. self-other)	–	–	–	–	–	–	–	–	–	–
Outcome variables										
2. T1 negative attitudes toward prescription opioids	0.08	–	–	–	–	–	–	–	–	–
3. T2 negative attitudes	0.42**	0.57**	–	–	–	–	–	–	–	–
4. T1 behavioral intentions	0.29*	0.44**	0.54**	–	–	–	–	–	–	–
5. T2 behavioral intentions	0.49**	0.64**	0.75**	0.72**	–	–	–	–	–	–
Mediators										
6. Fear	0.27*	0.26*	0.31*	0.38**	0.34*	–	–	–	–	–
7. Anticipated guilt	0.24*	0.38**	0.41**	0.40**	0.51**	0.38**	–	–	–	–

(*continued*)

Table 7.1 (continued)

Variables	*V1*	*V2*	*V3*	*V4*	*V5*	*V6*	*V7*	*V8*	*V9*	*V10*
Control variables										
8. Gender (male =1)	−0.19	−0.17	0.05	−0.16	−0.12	0.09	−0.09	–	–	–
9. Race (white =1)	0.09	0.12	−0.12	0.06	−0.10	0.12	0.14	−0.22	–	–
10. Prior exposure to anti-opioid messages	0.22	−0.01	0.19	0.19	0.20	0.22	−0.03	0.10	−0.12	–
11. Past misuse of opioids	0.07	−0.14	0.27	−0.29*	−0.01	−0.04	−0.10	0.16	−0.21	0.18

Notes: * $p<0.05$; ** $p<0.01$

7.4.4 *Data Analysis*

Independent t-tests were first conducted to examine whether there were any significant differences between participants completing only the first stage of the study and those completing both stages in terms of the control variables, mediators, and T1 outcome variables. The analyses found that white (vs. non-white) participants were more likely to complete both stages. Hence, race was also controlled in analyses involving the second stage.

Manipulation check was conducted using independent t-tests with reference focus as the grouping variable. To test the impacts of the reference focus (self vs. self-other) on mediators and T1 and T2 outcome variables, a series of analyses of covariance (ANCOVA) were conducted. After this, mixed-design ANCOVAs—with reference focus as a between-subjects factor and delay of assessment a within-subjects factor—were used to test whether the passage of time affected the impacts of the reference focus. The mediating roles of fear and anticipated guilt were examined using PROCESS, an SPSS macro (Hayes 2013). The macro uses a bootstrapping approach to estimate indirect effects; a significant indirect effect is indicated by a 95% bias-corrected confidence interval (BcCI) excluding zero.

7.5 Results

7.5.1 *Manipulation Check*

Participants who read the self-other-focused risk narratives (M_{first} = 5.71, *SD* = 1.52) were more likely than those who read the self-focused narratives (M_{third} = 4.38; *SD* = 1.66) to agree that the story highlighted the negative impacts of misusing prescription opioids on the family members of those who misused them ($t = 3.65$; $p < 0.001$). But the two groups were equally likely to agree that the story they read focused on the negative impacts of misusing prescription opioids on those who misused them (M_{self} = 5.36; *SD* = 1.56; $M_{self\text{-}other}$ = 5.63; *SD* = 1.34; $t = 0.82$; $p = 0.42$). Thus, the reference focus manipulation was successful.

7.5.2 *The Immediate and Delayed Attitudinal and Behavioral Impacts*

Although the self-focused versus self-other-focused risk narratives had no statistically significant immediate impact on negative attitudes toward prescription opioids (M_{self}= 5.49; *SD* = 1.28; $M_{self\text{-}other}$= 5.26; *SD* = 1.47; F [1,

72] = 0.26, $p = 0.61$), it had a significant positive delayed impact on the attitudes (M_{self}= 5.54, *SD* = 1.12; $M_{self\text{-}other}$= 4.18; *SD* = 1.81; F [1, 47] = 7.81, $p < 0.01$). Moreover, the self-focused narratives had significant positive immediate (M_{self} = 6.21; *SD* = 1.04; $M_{self\text{-}other}$ = 5.51; *SD* = 1.31; F [1, 71] = 5.28, $p < 0.05$) and delayed impacts (M_{self} = 6.35; *SD* = 0.81; $M_{self\text{-}other}$= 5.01; *SD* = 1.52; F [1, 47] = 11.28, $p < 0.01$) on intentions to avoid (mis)using prescription opioids. These findings partly supported the predictions that exposure to self-focused versus self-other-focused anti-prescription opioid risk narratives would increase negative attitudes toward prescription opioids (H1a) and intentions to avoid (mis)using the drugs (H1b) immediately after the exposure.

As for the impact of delay of assessment, there was no significant impact of the delay on attitudes toward prescription opioids (M_{T1} = 5.22; *SD* = 1.52; M_{T2} = 4.90; *SD* = 1.62; F [1, 47] = 3.81, $p = 0.06$). The analysis, however, detected a significant main effect of the reference focus (self vs. self-other; F [1, 47] = 6.16, $p < 0.05$) that was qualified by a significant interaction effect between the reference focus and the delay (F [1, 47] = 4.16; $p < 0.05$). The interaction effect was driven by the fact that the negative attitudes toward prescription opioids decreased among participants in the self-other-focused condition between T1 and T2 assessment but changed little among those in the self-focused condition (see Fig. 7.1).

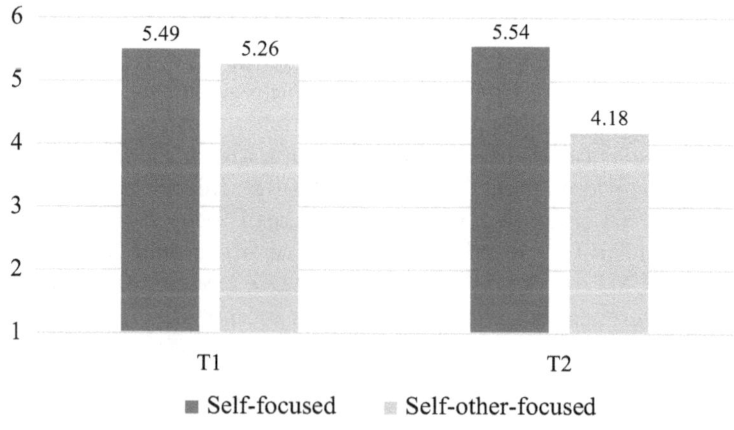

Fig. 7.1 The interaction effect of reference focus and delay of assessment on negative attitudes toward prescription opioids

Along the same lines, delay of assessment had no significant impact on intentions to avoid (mis)using prescription opioids ($M_{T1} = 5.75$, $SD = 1.43$; $M_{T2} = 5.72$; $SD = 1.36$; $F [1, 47] = 1.47$, $p = 0.23$). The analysis, however, found a significant main effect of the reference focus (self vs. self-other; $F [1, 47] = 17.03$, $p < 0.001$) but not a significant interaction effect between the reference focus and the delay of assessment ($F [1, 47] = 0.34$, $p = 0.56$). These findings indicated that the predicted positive attitudinal and behavioral impacts of exposure to the self-focused (vs. self-other-focused) anti-prescription opioid risk narratives did not diminish after a period of time (RQ1).

7.5.3 *The Mediating Roles of Fear and Anticipated Guilt*

As predicted, exposure to the self-focused (vs. self-other-focused) narratives aroused greater fear ($M_{self} = 3.59$; $SD = 1.92$; $M_{self\text{-}other} = 2.62$; $SD = 1.61$; $F [1, 71] = 5.14$, $p < 0.05$), supporting the prediction that exposure to self-focused vs. self-other-focused anti-prescription opioid risk narratives would induce greater fear immediately after the exposure (H2). Although the main effect analysis did not find the predicted significant immediate positive impact of the reference focus (self vs. self-other) on negative attitudes toward prescription opioids, the reference focus may still have significant indirect effects on the attitudes via the proposed mediators (Hayes 2013). Indeed, indirect effect analyses found that the reference focus had indirect positive impacts on T1 negative attitudes toward prescription opioids (Effect = 0.20; $p < 0.05$) and T1 intentions to avoid (mis)using the drugs (Effect = 0.19; $p < 0.05$; see Table 7.2) via increased fear. These findings partly supported the predictions that the immediate positive attitudinal (H3a) and behavioral impacts (H3b) of exposure to self-focused versus self-other-focused anti-prescription opioid risk narratives would be (partly) explained by increased fear.

Also as anticipated, exposure to the self-focused (vs. self-other-focused) narratives aroused greater anticipated guilt ($M_{self} = 5.08$; $SD = 2.08$; $M_{self\text{-}other} = 4.10$; $SD = 2.29$; $F [1, 71] = 4.23$; $p < 0.05$), lending support to the hypothesis that exposure to self-focused vs. self-other-focused anti-prescription opioid risk narratives would arouse greater anticipated guilt immediately after the exposure (H4). Indirect effect analyses showed that the reference focus had indirect positive impacts on T1 attitudes (Effect = 0.26; $p < 0.05$) and T1 behavioral intentions (Effect = 0.22; $p < 0.05$) via increased anticipated guilt, which partly supported the predictions that the immediate positive attitudinal (H5a) and behavioral impacts (H5b) of

Table 7.2 Results of indirect effect analyses

Indirect effects	*Effect*	*95% BcCI*
Reference focus (self vs. self-other)➔fear➔T1 negative attitudes	0.20*	0.01, 0.50
Reference focus➔fear➔T1 behavioral intentions	0.19*	0.03, 0.46
Reference focus➔anticipated guilt➔T1 attitudes	0.26*	0.01, 0.62
Reference focus➔anticipated guilt➔T1 intentions	0.22*	0.01, 0.53
Reference focus➔fear➔T2 attitudes	0.25	−0.06, 0.79
Reference focus➔fear➔T2 intentions	0.20	−0.04, 0.62
Reference focus➔anticipated guilt➔T2 attitudes	0.50*	0.03, 1.19
Reference focus➔anticipated guilt➔T2 intentions	0.54*	0.08, 1.18
Direct effects	*Effect*	*95% BcCI*
Reference focus➔(fear)➔T1 attitudes	−0.03	−0.70, 0.63
Reference focus➔(fear)➔T1 intentions	0.43	−0.10, 0.95
Reference focus➔(anticipated guilt)➔T1 attitudes	−0.09	−0.73, 0.54
Reference focus➔(anticipated guilt)➔T1 intentions	0.40	−0.11, 0.90
Reference focus➔(fear)➔T2 attitudes	1.07*	0.07, 2.07
Reference focus➔(fear)➔T2 intentions	1.11*	0.28, 1.94
Reference focus➔(anticipated guilt)➔T2 attitudes	0.82	−0.17, 1.82
Reference focus➔(anticipated guilt)➔T2 intentions	0.77	−0.01, 1.55

Notes: Direct effects indicate the relationships between the reference focus (self vs. self-other), on one hand, and negative attitudes toward prescription opioids and intentions to avoid (mis)using the drugs, on the other hand, while controlling the influence of the mediator being tested. All the control variables in ANCOVAs were included in the direct and indirect effect analyses

* $p < 0.05$

exposure to self-focused versus self-other-focused anti-prescription opioid risk narratives would be (partly) explained by increased anticipated guilt.

Given that the indirect effect analyses with either fear or anticipated guilt as the mediator found that both explained the immediate attitudinal and behavioral impacts of the reference focus, additional indirect effect analyses were conducted to test both mediators simultaneously. The analyses found that when both mediators were included in the analyses, only the indirect attitudinal and behavioral impacts of the reference focus via anticipated guilt were statistically significant (T1 attitude, Effect = 0.23; $p < 0.05$; T1 intentions, Effect = 0.18; $p < 0.05$) and those via fear were no longer significant (T1 attitude, Effect = 0.11; $p > 0.05$; T1 intentions, Effect = 0.12; $p > 0.05$).

As for the roles of fear and anticipated guilt aroused immediately after exposure to the narratives in explaining the delayed attitudinal and behavioral impacts of the reference focus, the analyses found that fear did not explain the delayed impacts (T2 attitude, Effect = 0.25; $p > 0.05$; T2 intentions, Effect = 0.20; $p > 0.05$) but anticipated guilt did (T2 attitude, Effect = 0.50; $p < 0.05$; T2 intentions, Effect = 0.54; $p < 0.05$). These findings suggested that anticipated guilt aroused immediately after exposure to the self-focused versus self-other-focused anti-prescription opioid risk narratives explained the delayed positive attitudinal and behavioral impacts of the reference focus (RQ3) but the fear aroused immediately after the exposure did not (RQ2).

7.6 Discussion

This study explored the immediate and delayed impacts of the reference focus (self vs. self-other) of anti-prescription opioid risk narratives on negative attitudes toward prescription opioids and intentions to avoid (mis) using the drugs while considering the mediating roles of fear and anticipated guilt. It found that exposure to self-focused (vs. self-other-focused) narratives aroused greater fear and anticipated guilt and increased intentions to avoid (mis)using prescription opioids immediately after the exposure. It also detected delayed positive attitudinal and behavioral impacts of exposure to self-focused narratives about two weeks after the exposure. The observed immediate and delayed attitudinal and behavioral impacts of the reference focus were mainly explained by anticipated guilt aroused immediately after the exposure.

7.6.1 Theoretical Implications

This study was the first to investigate the immediate and delayed attitudinal and behavioral impacts of the reference focus of risk narratives in the context of health campaigns and among the first to explore the role of emotions in explaining the impacts of the reference focus of persuasive messages. By examining the mediating roles of fear and anticipated guilt at the same time, this study answered the call for exploration of the influence of multiple emotions aroused simultaneously by persuasive appeals on the effectiveness of such appeals (Carcioppolo et al. 2017, 454). Its findings advance our understanding of the influence of reference focus on persuasion.

The observed immediate and delayed positive attitudinal and behavioral impacts of the self-focused (vs. self-other-focused) risk narratives support the argument that unlike non-narrative messages that highlight the negative impacts of incompliance on the self, their narrative counterparts are unlikely to induce negative reactions (e.g., counterarguing and psychological reactance) because of narratives' ability to overcome resistance to persuasion (Moyer-Guse and Nabi 2010; Ratcliff and Sun 2020). The observed impacts also lend support to CLT (Trope and Liberman 2010), which suggests that self-focused risks are perceived to be psychologically closer than other-focused risks. As a result, risks involving the self are represented in more specific and concrete terms than those involving both the self and others, as the latter should be represented in mixed concrete and abstract terms. The more concrete representation of self-focused risks in turn increases risk perceptions and recommendation compliance (Chandran and Menon 2004). Furthermore, the findings are consistent with the notion that psychological distance-related factors (e.g., social distance in the case of this study) can be used to manipulate the concreteness of risk communication and therefore influence persuasion (Chandran and Menon 2004; Yang and McAllister 2020).

Besides detecting the delayed positive attitudinal and behavioral impacts of exposure to self-focused (vs. self-other-focused) risk narratives, this study also found that the attitudinal impact of the self-focused risk narratives became statistically significant over time because the negative attitudes toward prescription opioids declined over time among participants in the self-other-focused condition but remained unchanged among those in the self-focused condition. Moreover, the strength of the significant positive behavioral impact of the self-focused narratives did not diminish over time. These findings indicate that self-focused risk narratives can have long-lasting impacts, and under some circumstances their impacts may be less likely to dwindle over time than risk narratives adopting a different reference focus.

As for the mediating role of emotions, this study found that exposure to self-focused (vs. self-other-focused) risk narratives had immediate indirect positive attitudinal and behavioral impacts via fear and anticipated guilt when each mediator was tested separately. However, when both mediators were tested simultaneously, only the indirect impacts through anticipated guilt were still statistically significant. Anticipated guilt, not fear, was also found to explain the delayed positive attitudinal and behavioral impacts of exposure to self-focused narratives. These findings suggest that emotions play an important role in explaining the influence of the reference focus of risk narratives and that changing the reference focus of such narratives can shape the experience of multiple emotions on the part of message receivers. The findings also heighten the importance of investigating the influence of multiple emotions aroused simultaneously by persuasive appeals on their effectiveness (Carcioppolo et al. 2017, 454) and support the argument that emotions often serve as motivators for changes (Yang and McAllister 2020). Beyond this, these findings are consistent with earlier research suggesting that fear and anticipated guilt are positive predictors of persuasion (White and Albarracin 2018; O'Keefe 2002; Cao 2023, 2024). More importantly, the findings indicate the relative contribution of two emotions—fear and anticipated guilt—to the impacts of the reference focus (self vs. self-other) of risk narratives.

7.6.2 *Practical Implications*

By showing that self-focused (vs. self-other-focused) anti-prescription opioid risk narratives produced desired attitudinal and behavioral impacts that lasted over time among a convenience sample of college students, my findings indicate that using self-focused risk narratives may be an effective strategy to discourage risky behaviors, including (mis)using prescription opioids, among people—especially young people, a demographic group that is most likely to engage in risky behaviors and resist the influence of health messages (Levy 2019, 3). Moreover, the observation that anticipated guilt explained the immediate and delayed attitudinal and behavioral impacts of the reference focus of risk narratives suggests that health messages that arouse anticipated guilt may exert not only immediate but also long-lasting influence on message receivers. Hence, campaign designers may consider appealing to anticipated guilt to increase the effectiveness of their messages.

Most participants of this study (94%) reported no experience of misusing prescription opioids. As a result, self-focused (vs. self-other-focused) anti-prescription opioid risk narratives aroused greater anticipated guilt in this study, as anticipated guilt is experienced when individuals imagine or anticipate their violation of personal, societal, and/or moral standards (Lindsey 2005, 455; Carcioppolo et al. 2017, 438). Such narratives likely elicit reactive guilt (an emotional state experienced after people have violated personal, societal, and/or moral standards; Lazarus 1991 cited in Cao 2024, 252) among people who have the experience of misusing prescription opioids. Because reactive guilt is more likely than anticipated guilt to trigger negative reactions to persuasive messages (Renner et al. 2013), designers of anti-prescription opioid campaigns need to be mindful of the target audience's overall experience with prescription opioids when attempting to deploy guilt appeals (e.g., self-focused risk narratives).

7.6.3 *Strengths, Limitations, and Future Research*

This study has several strengths and weaknesses. Beginning with the strengths, this study used more than one story to investigate the impacts of the reference focus of risk narratives, which increased my confidence that the findings were not driven by the idiosyncrasies of one story. The experimental nature of the study enabled me to ascertain causal relationships between the reference focus, on one hand, and the mediators and outcome variables under study, on the other hand. Moreover, narratives used in this study were created based on real stories of people with OUD, which increased the external validity of my findings.

Turning to limitations, this study was conducted among a convenience sample of college students. Future research may use a representative sample of American (young) adults to retest the impacts observed here. Given that most participants of this study had no experience of misusing prescription opioids, further research may test the impacts of the reference focus of anti-prescription opioid risk narratives among people with such experience. Moreover, this study used behavioral intentions to test the behavioral impact of the reference focus. Future research may test the influence of the reference focus on actual behavior.

The risk narratives used in this study were presented in the form of testimonials and delivered via print media. Given that such narratives can be presented in other forms (e.g., anecdotes) and are often delivered via multiple modalities (e.g., CDC's Rx Awareness campaign 2021), future research may examine whether my findings extend to other forms of risk narratives and other modalities. This study tested the impacts of the reference focus of risk narratives in the context of anti-prescription opioid campaigns. Future studies may explore whether my findings extend to other risky behaviors, given that research has shown that the impacts of narratives vary depending upon the behavior being promoted (Graaf et al. 2016, 91).

This study only tested the roles of two emotions—fear and anticipated guilt—in explaining the impacts of the reference focus of risk narratives; further studies may consider expanding the investigation to include other emotions (e.g., anger). Such studies may also simultaneously examine the contribution of affective and cognitive factors to the influence of the reference focus of persuasive messages, as cognitive factors (e.g., message elaboration and processing fluency) have been found to explain the impacts of the reference focus of non-narrative messages (Hong and Hashimoto 2023; Huang and Li 2023).

Despite these limitations, this study was the first to investigate the immediate and delayed impacts of the reference focus of risk narratives and among the first to explore the role of emotions in explaining the influence of the reference focus of persuasive appeals. Its findings not only contribute to our understanding of the influence of the reference focus of persuasive messages but also provide guidance in the design of effective public health campaigns.

Appendix: Stories Used in the Study

Self-Focused Version of Story 1

"It all started with a back injury. My doctor prescribed me an opioid pain medication that lasted a lot longer than the pain itself. At the time, I didn't understand the danger of the drug. *How can I get addicted? I get them from my doctor.* Within only a few months, I became completely addicted. I have suffered through opioid withdrawals so badly that I thought I was dying. Now all I'm concerned about is finding more pills and more prescription opioids to avoid the withdrawals. As I'm watching my friends dying of drug overdoses, I know I'm on the same path. I'm really scared and don't want to live like this anymore, but I'm too ashamed to ask for help."

—Steve, died of an opioid overdose at 24

Self-Other-Focused Version of Story 1

"My son, Steve, was first prescribed opioids after hurting his back. Within only a few months, he changed into another person. I didn't know what was going on until I saw him lying on the floor, trembling, sick and crying. When he admitted his drug addiction to me, I was completely shocked. He told me he really wanted to get better but was too ashamed to ask for help. He died of a prescription opioid overdose three days later. He was due to start a treatment program the next day. That's the darkest day of my life. I'm not supposed to be the one to get his suit and tie and pick which sneakers I'm going to bury him in. I love and miss my son and forever will."

—Jenny whose son died of an opioid overdose at 24

Self-Focused Version of Story 2

"I used to have a good career and a beautiful family. But they were all taken away by prescription opioids. I was diagnosed with cancer and prescribed an opioid pain killer during the treatment. I never thought I would be addicted to a drug given by a doctor. I took the drug exactly as prescribed but still got addicted to it. My addiction changed me into this "other" person. When looking in the mirror, I don't recognize my reflection. I no longer am the girl I knew. The addiction stole everything from me. I wound up homeless. Every day I'm consumed by shame, guilt, and embarrassment. I really want to get better, but I'm too ashamed to ask for help."—Jessica

Self-Other-Focused Version of Story 2

"My daughter, Jessica, had a good career and a beautiful family. But prescription opioids changed all of it. She was prescribed an opioid pain medication during her cancer treatment. Soon she became addicted to the medication even though she was taking it exactly as prescribed. The addiction consumes every aspect of her life and has changed her into another person. It seems that nothing matters to her anymore. She has lost everything she had, become homeless, and even put her child in danger. No words can describe the despair of watching my beautiful daughter succumb to drug addiction. Now I'm raising my granddaughter. It's heartbreaking to comfort her and explain to her why Mama isn't coming home. This horrifying addiction has scarred my family forever."—Mary

References

Allara, Elias, Marica Ferri, Alessandra Bo, Antonio Gasparrini, and Fabrizio Faggiano. 2015. Are Mass-Media Campaigns Effective in Preventing Drug use? A Cochrane Systematic Review and Meta-Analysis. *BMJ Open* 5:e007449. https://doi.org/10.1136/bmjopen-2014-007449.

Antonetti, Paolo, Paul Baines, and Shailendra Jain. 2018. The Persuasiveness of Guilt Appeals Over Time: Pathways to Delayed Compliance. *Journal of Business Research* 90:14–25. https://doi.org/10.1016/j.jbusres.2018.03.030.

Banerjee, Smita C., and Kathryn Greene. 2012. Role of Transportation in the Persuasion Process: Cognitive and Affective Responses to Anti-Drug Narratives. *Journal of Health Communication* 17 (5): 564–581. https://doi.org/10.1080/10810730.2011.635779.

Beyer, Don. 2022. JEC Analysis Finds Opioid Epidemic Cost U.S. Nearly $1.5 Trillion in 2020. *The U.S. Congress Joint Economic Committee,* September 28. https://beyer.house.gov/news/documentsingle.aspx?DocumentID=5684.

Bigman, Cabral A., Rebekah H. Nagler, and K. Viswanath. 2016. Representation, Exemplification, and Risk: Resonance of Tobacco Graphic Health Warnings across Diverse Populations. *Health Communication* 31 (8): 974–987. https://doi.org/10.1080/10410236.2015.1026430.

Birkimer, John C., Philip L. Johnston, and Melissa M. Berry. 1993. Guilt and Help from Friends: Variables Related to Healthy Behavior. *Journal of Social Psychology* 133 (5): 683–692. https://doi.org/10.1080/00224545.1993.9713923.

Block, Lauren G. 2005. Self-Referenced Fear and Guilt Appeals: The Moderating Role of Self-Construal. *Journal of Applied Social Psychology* 35 (11): 2290–2309. https://doi.org/10.1111/j.1559-1816.2005.tb02103.x.

Brundage, Suzanne C., and Carol Levine. 2019. *The Ripple Effect: The Impact of the Opioid Epidemic on Children and Families.* http://addictionmedicineupdates.org/wp-content/uploads/2019/04/The-Ripple-Effect.pdf.

Cao, Xiaoxia. 2023. The Impact of the Reference Focus of Anti-Prescription Opioid Campaigns on Young Americans: The Roles of Anticipated Guilt and Psychological Reactance. *Atlantic Journal of Communication* 31 (4): 312–324. https://doi.org/10.1080/15456870.2022.2081691.

Cao, Xiaoxia. 2024. The Impacts of Narrative Perspectives of Anti-Prescription Opioid Campaigns: The Mediating Roles of Identification, Perceived Severity, and Anticipated Guilt. *Health Communication* 39 (2): 244–257. https://doi.org/10.1080/10410236.2022.2163110.

Carcioppolo, Nick, Cong Li, Elena V. Chudnovskaya, Rebecca Kharsa, Tyler Stephan, and Kelly Nickel. 2017. The Comparative Efficacy of a Hybrid Guilt-Fear Appeal and a Traditional Fear Appeal to Influence HPV Vaccination Intentions. *Communication Research* 44 (3): 437–458. https://doi.org/10.1177/0093650215616457.

Chandran, Sucharita, and Geeta Menon. 2004. When a Day Means More than a Year: Effects of Temporal Framing on Judgments of Health Risk. *Journal of Consumer Research* 31 (2): 375–389. https://doi.org/10.1086/422116.

Chen, Meng, and Robert A. Bell. 2022. A Meta-Analysis of the Impact of Point of View on Narrative Processing and Persuasion in Health Messaging. *Psychology & Health* 37 (5): 545–562. https://doi.org/10.1080/08870446.2021.1894331.

Fishbein, Martin, and Icek Ajzen. 2009. *Predicting and Changing Behavior: The Reasoned Action Approach.* Psychological Press.

Frakt, Austin, and Keith Humphreys. 2017. Just Say No to Opioids? Ads Could Actually Make Things Worse. *New York Times*, November 1. https://www.nytimes.com/2017/11/01/upshot/why-advertising-is-a-poor-choice-to-tackle-the-opioid-crisis.html.

Frank, Lily E., and Saskia K. Nagel. 2017. Addiction and Moralization: The Role of the Underlying Model Addiction. *Neuroethics* 10 (1): 129–139. https://doi.org/10.1007/s12152-017-9307-x.

Gardner, Liz, and Glenn Leshner. 2016. The Role of Narrative and Other-Referencing in Attenuating Psychological Reactance to Diabetes Self-Care Messages. *Health Communication* 31 (6): 738–751. https://doi.org/10.1080/10410236.2014.993498.

Graaf, Anneke de, Jose Sanders, and Hans Hoeken. 2016. Characteristics of Narrative Interventions and Health Effects: A Review of the Content, Form, and Context of Narratives in Health-Related Narrative Persuasion Research. *Review of Communication Research* 4:88–131. https://rcommunicationr.org/index.php/rcr/article/view/24.

Green, Melanie C., and Timothy C. Brock. 2000. The Role of Transportation in the Persuasiveness of Public Narratives. *Journal of Personality and Social Psychology* 79 (5): 701–721. https://doi.org/10.1037/0022-3514.79.5.701.

Han, Da Hee, Adam Duhachek, and Nidhi Agrawal. 2014. Emotions Shape Decisions through Construal Level: The Case of Guilt and Shame. *Journal of Consumer Research* 41 (4): 1047–1064. https://doi.org/10.1086/678300.

Hayes, Andrew F. 2013. *Introduction to Mediation, Moderation, and Conditional Process Analysis: A Regression-Based Approach*. The Guilford Press.

Hong, Yangsun, and Mika Hashimoto. 2023. I Will Get Myself Vaccinated for Others: The Interplay of Message Frame, Reference Point, and Perceived Risk on Intention for Covid-19 Vaccine. *Health Communication* 38 (4): 813–823. https://doi.org/10.1080/10410236.2021.1978668.

Huang, Guanxiong, and Kang Li. 2023. Get Vaccinated for Loved Ones: Effects of Self-Other Appeal and Message Framing in Promoting HPV Vaccination among Heterosexual Young Men. *Health Communication* 38 (2): 381–393. https://doi.org/10.1080/10410236.2021.1953728.

Kim, Hye Kyung, and Tae Kyoung Lee. 2018. Curious or Afraid of Using Study Drugs? The Effects of Self-Referent Thoughts and Identification on Anticipated Affect. *International Journal of Communication* 12:2421–2442. 1932–8036/20180005.

Kreuter, Matthew W., Melanie C. Green, Joseph N. Cappella, et al. 2007. Narrative Communication in Cancer Prevention and Control: A Framework to Guide Research and Application. *Annals of Behavioral Medicine* 33 (3): 221–235. https://doi.org/10.1007/BF02879904.

Levy, Sharon. 2019. Youth and Opioid Epidemic. *Pediatrics* 143 (2): e2018–e2753. https://doi.org/10.1542/peds.2018-2752.

Li, Kang, and Nora Rifon. 2017. The Effects of Message Framing and Reference Points of Public Service Announcements on Bystander Intervention in College Students' Binge-Drinking. In *Advances in Advertising Research*, edited by

Geroge Christodoulides and Anastasia Stathopoulou, vol. VII. and Martin Eisend. European Advertising Academy.

Lindsey, Lisa L. Massi. 2005. Anticipated Guilt as Behavioral Motivation: An Examination of Appeals to Help Unknown Others through Bone Marrow Donation. *Human Communication Research* 31 (4): 453–481. https://doi.org/10.1111/j.1468-2958.2005.tb00879.x.

Loroz, Peggy S. 2007. The Interaction of Message Frames and Reference Points in Prosocial Persuasive Appeals. *Psychology & Marketing* 24 (11): 1001–1023. https://doi.org/10.1002/mar.20193.

Ma, Haijing, and Claude H. Miller. 2021. The Effects of Agency Assignment and Reference Point on Responses to Covid-19 Messages. *Health Communication* 36 (1): 59–73. https://doi.org/10.1080/10410236.2020.1848066.

Meadows, Cui Zhang. 2020. The Effects of Fear Appeals and Message Format on Promoting Skin Cancer Prevention Behaviors among College Students. *Societies* 10 (1): 21. https://doi.org/10.3390/soc10010021.

Moyer-Guse, Emily, and Robin L. Nabi. 2010. Explaining the Effects of Narrative in an Entertainment Television Program: Overcoming Resistance to Persuasion. *Human Communication Research* 36 (1): 26–52. https://doi.org/10.1111/j.1468-2958.2009.01367.x.

National Center for Health Statistics. 2024. *Drug Overdoses.* July 23. https://www.cdc.gov/nchs/fastats/drug-overdoses.htm.

National Institute on Drug Abuse. 2022. *Overdose Death Rates.* January 20. https://nida.nih.gov/research-topics/trends-statistics/overdose-death-rates.

National Safety Council. 2022. *Drug Overdoses.* https://injuryfacts.nsc.org/home-and-community/safety-topics/drugoverdoses/#:~:text=The%20 25%2D%20to% 2034%2Dage,and%20older%20is%20still%20growing.

O'Keefe, Daniel J. 2002. Guilt as a Mechanism of Persuasion. In *The Persuasion Handbook: Developments in Theory and Practice*, edited by Jame Price Dillard and Lijiang Shen. Sage.

Oh, Sang-Hwa, Hye-Jin Paek, and Thomas Hove. 2015. Cognitive and Emotional Dimensions of Perceived Risk Characteristics, Genre-Specific Media Effects, and Risk Perceptions: The Case of H1N1 Influenza in South Korea. *Asian Journal of Communication* 25 (1): 14–32. https://doi.org/10.1080/01292986.2014.989240.

Public Broadcasting Service. 2022. *Frontline: Heron & Opioid Addiction, in Your Own Words.* https://www.pbs.org/wgbh/frontline/interactive/heroin-stories/theme/friends-and-family.html.

Ratcliff, Chelsea L., and Ye Sun. 2020. Overcoming Resistance through Narratives: Findings from a Meta-Analytic Review. *Human Communication Research* 46 (4): 412–443. https://doi.org/10.1093/hcr/hqz017.

Renner, Simone, Jörg Lindenmeier, Dieter K. Tscheulin, and Florian Drevs. 2013. Guilt Appeals and Prosocial Behavior: An Experimental Analysis of the Effects of Anticipatory versus Reactive Guilt Appeals on the Effectiveness of Blood

Donor Appeals. *Journal of Nonprofit & Public Sector Marketing* 25 (3): 237–255. https://doi.org/10.1080/10495142.2013.816595.
Richard, Rene, Joop van der Pligt, and Nanne de Vries. 1996. Anticipated Affect and Behavioral Choice. *Basic and Applied Social Psychology* 18 (2): 111–129. https://doi.org/10.1207/s15324834basp1802_1.
Shen, Fuyuan, Vivian C. Sheer, and Ruobing Li. 2015. Impact of Narratives on Persuasion in Health Communication: A Meta-Analysis. *Journal of Advertising* 44 (2): 105–113. https://doi.org/10.1080/00913367.2015.1018467.
Staunton, Thomas V., Eusebio M. Alvaro, and Benjamin D. Rosenberg. 2022. A Case for Directives: Strategies for Enhancing Clarity While Mitigating Reactance. *Current Psychology* 41:611–621. https://doi.org/10.1007/s12144-019-00588-0.
Tannenbaum, Melaine B., Justin Hepler, Rick S. Zimmerman, et al. 2015. Appealing to Fear: A Meta-Analysis of Fear Appeal Effectiveness and Theories. *Psychological Bulletin* 141 (6): 1178–1204. https://doi.org/10.1037/a0039729.
Trope, Yaacov, and Nira Liberman. 2010. Construal Level Theory of Psychological Distance. *Psychological Review* 117 (2): 440–463. https://doi.org/10.1037/a0018963.
Turner, Monique Mitchell. 2017. Using Guilt to Motivate Individuals to Adopt Healthy Habits. In *Oxford Encyclopedia of Communication*, edited by Jon Nussbaum. Oxford.
U.S. Centers for Disease Control and Prevention. 2021. *Rx Awareness*. https://www.cdc.gov/rxawareness/index.html.
White, Benjamin X., and Dolores Albarracin. 2018. Investigating Belief Falsehood. Fear Appeals Do Change Behavior in Experimental Laboratory Studies. A Commentary on Kok et al. (2018). *Health Psychology Review* 12 (2): 147–150. https://doi.org/10.1080/17437199.2018.1448292.
Witte, Kim. 1992. Putting the Fear Back into Fear Appeals: The Extended Parallel Process Model. *Communication Monographs* 59 (4): 225–249. https://doi.org/10.1080/03637759209376276.
Witte, Kim, and Mike Allen. 2000. A Meta-Analysis of Fear Appeals: Implications for Effective Public Health Campaigns. *Health Education & Behavior* 27 (5): 591–615. https://doi.org/10.1177/109019810002700506.
Wong, Norman C. H., Kylie J. Harrison, and Lindsey A. Harvell. 2015. Reactance and Public Health Messages: The Unintended Dangers of Anti-Tobacco PSAs. *Studies in Media and Communication* 3 (2): 72–82. https://doi.org/10.11114/smc.v3i2.1022.
Xu, Jie, and Xiaoxia Cao. 2020. Young Adults' (Mis)use of Prescription Opioid Drugs: An Exploratory Study. *Health Communication* 35 (11): 1407–1414. https://doi.org/10.1080/10410236.2019.1636343.
Yang, Janet Z., and C. A. S. S. McAllister. 2020. Closer to the Heart, Closer to the Mind: Using Psychological Distance to Communicate a Measles Outbreak. *Journal of Health Communication* 25 (11): 895–902. https://doi.org/10.1080/10810730.2020.1851822.

CHAPTER 8

Bridging Knowledge and Practice: Collaborative Academic Detailing During the Opioid Crisis

Meghan N. Breckling and *Leah R. Tobey-Moore*

8.1 The Link Between Pain Management and the Opioid Epidemic

Opioid overprescribing has resulted in increased misuse even among people without an opioid prescription. The opioid overdose crisis has unfolded in three waves: prescription opioid deaths in the 1990s, a rise in heroin deaths beginning in 2010, and, since 2013, a surge in deaths from synthetic opioids such as illicit fentanyl and its analogs (Centers for Disease Control and Prevention 2025). In the 2023 National Survey on Drug Use and Health, 8.2 million people aged 12 or older reported misusing

M. N. Breckling (✉)
Department of Pharmacy Practice, University of Arkansas for Medical Sciences, Little Rock, AR, USA
e-mail: MNBreckling@uams.edu

L. R. Tobey-Moore
Department of Psychiatry, University of Arkansas for Medical Sciences, Little Rock, AR, USA
e-mail: LTobeymoore@uams.edu

X. Cao (ed.), *Fighting the Opioid Crisis with Communication*,
https://doi.org/10.1007/978-3-032-31162-7_8

prescription pain relievers, and about 45% of these respondents said that their opioids were prescribed by a doctor (Substance Abuse and Mental Health Services Administration 2024). In 2023, approximately 105,000 people died from drug overdoses, and nearly 80,000 (76%) of those deaths involved an opioid (Centers for Disease Control and Prevention 2025). To address opioid overprescribing and decrease overdose deaths, the Centers for Disease Control and Prevention (CDC) released guidelines for healthcare providers with recommendations for safer opioid prescribing and pain management.

The first version of the *Guideline for Prescribing Opioids for Chronic Pain* was released by the CDC in 2016 (Dowell et al. 2016). The primary intention of these guidelines was to help primary care clinicians weigh the benefits and risks of opioid treatment for chronic pain. Following the release, there was a major reduction in overall and potentially high-risk prescribing of opioids and an increase in the prescribing of non-opioid pain medications. In response to the guidelines, many states introduced new laws, regulations, and policies; however, these policies were enforced too strictly or deviated from the intended use of the recommendations. Some misapplications included inflexible dosage and duration thresholds for opioids, which contributed to patient harm, untreated pain conditions, dangerous abrupt discontinuations leading to acute withdrawal symptoms, psychological distress, and even suicidal ideation and behavior for some people (Dowell et al. 2022). These harmful outcomes highlighted the need for an updated guideline to emphasize the importance of flexible, individualized, and patient-centered pain management, including new evidence-based treatment options for various types of pain and safe opioid tapering practices.

The CDC released an updated version in 2022 titled the *Clinical Practice Guideline for Prescribing Opioids for Pain* (Dowell et al. 2022) that focused on (1) safer initiation of opioid treatment, (2) selecting opioids and dosages, (3) determining the duration of initial prescriptions and follow-up, and (4) assessing and mitigating opioid-related risks. These guidelines aim to improve clinician-patient communication, enhance treatment safety and effectiveness, improve pain management and quality of life, and reduce risks like opioid use disorder, overdose, and death. The new version expanded the scope of the guidelines by including all clinicians who are treating acute, subacute, and chronic pain while it also encourages more flexibility in recommendations to balance the risks and benefits of opioid treatments for individual patients. The emphasis on non-opioid treatment is still present in the 2022 updates, but there is also mention that opioids may be an appropriate treatment in specific cases. Based on these guidelines, opioid treatment is not recommended as first-line therapy for many common acute pain conditions (e.g., low back pain, musculoskeletal injuries, pain related to minor surgeries, with a duration of less than one month). It should be reserved for acute pain related to severe traumatic injuries, including crush injuries and burns. For treating chronic pain (pain with a duration greater than three months), the guidelines recommend avoiding long-term use of prescription opioids based on insufficient evidence of the benefits of their use and the existence of evidence showing the increased risk for overdose and opioid misuse (Mackey et al. 2019).

A major change in the 2022 guideline was the removal of the rigid morphine milligram equivalent (MME) limits, which is a standard measure used to compare the potency of different opioid medications by converting dosages into an equivalent amount of morphine to help prescribers assess opioid strength, monitor dosing, and reduce overall risk. The 2016 guidelines set a specific MME threshold at cautioning against dosing opioids at 50 MME and above and avoiding doses 90 MME and above, when possible, whereas the 2022 guidelines instead advise clinicians to use clinical judgment and carefully assess the benefits and risks of opioid treatment for each patient. This change in recommendation was likely due to the misapplication of the 2016 guidelines in various laws and policies that led to the unsafe and even harmful abrupt discontinuation of opioid treatment for many patients due to strictly enforced MME limitations. To combat these harmful consequences, the new 2022 guidelines stress the risks of rapidly tapering opioids and strongly recommend gradual, patient-centered tapering plans to avoid withdrawal and harm.

Additional changes in the updated 2022 guidelines included a transition from the 2016 framework, which placed strict three-to-seven day limitations on acute opioid prescriptions and sought to avoid long-term opioid use, to an approach with no strict duration limits, instead advising healthcare providers to prescribe only as long as medically necessary for the specific condition and to regularly reassess the need for continued use. The 2016 guidelines strongly discouraged the co-prescribing of opioids and benzodiazepines, whereas the updated 2022 version advises caution and acknowledges that some patients may require both medications, with close monitoring by their provider. Another significant change in the new guidelines was the addition of risk mitigation recommendations, including naloxone prescribing, prevention and screening for opioid use disorder, and prescribing approved medications for this condition when appropriate. Overall, the new updated 2022 guidelines stress the importance of more flexibility with recommendations, individualized patient care, shared decision-making, and balancing the risks and benefits of various pain treatments when making clinical decisions. The guidelines deliver a comprehensive framework for opioid prescribing, emphasizing the patient's quality of life, patient safety, and risk mitigation. By applying these recommendations through patient-centered care, healthcare practitioners can reduce the risks of opioid use disorder and opioid overdose through safer prescribing and patient education, all while still addressing patients' chronic pain needs.

8.1.1 *Safer Opioid Prescribing: Barriers, Supports, and Solutions*

Although the 2022 CDC guidelines aim to restore clinical judgment and support individualized patient care, implementation of recommendations by healthcare professionals remains challenging due to various regulatory barriers, the lingering consequences of misapplying the 2016 guidelines, and limited access to recommended evidence-based non-opioid pain management options. Many clinicians remain hesitant to prescribe opioids, even when medically appropriate, because of systemic, legal, and practical concerns. The misapplication of the 2016 guidelines fostered a climate of caution, with providers fearing regulatory repercussions. While the 2022 update removed strict dosage thresholds, many state laws and insurance policies still enforce opioid dosing limits or require prior authorizations, adding further complexity and obstacless to treatment when necessary. Concerns about the Drug Enforcement Administration (DEA) scrutiny, medical board discipline, and malpractice liability continue to discourage appropriate opioid prescribing. Additionally, inconsistent adoption of prescribing policies across healthcare systems (driven by variations in state regulations, insurance coverage, and pharmacy practices) makes it difficult for clinicians to apply a patient-centered approach to pain treatment (U.S. Food and Drug Administration 2020).

While the 2022 guidelines eliminated strict dose limits to encourage individualized care, the lack of clear thresholds has introduced some uncertainty for clinicians trying to balance effective pain relief with safe and responsible prescribing. Patients may also struggle to trust healthcare providers who previously implemented abrupt opioid tapers, which in some cases led to uncomfortable withdrawal symptoms, worsened pain, or even the transition to dangerous illicit opioids, raising the risk of opioid use disorder and overdose (U.S. Food and Drug Administration 2019). Rebuilding patient trust and determining how to reintroduce appropriate pain treatments remain significant challenges. Additionally, stigma surrounding opioid prescribing continues to impact patient care, as many providers fear the label of "over-prescribers" of opioids. Even when opioids are prescribed for indicated conditions, patients and prescribers often encounter challenges with access at the pharmacy level due to evolving insurance and organizational policies aimed at addressing the opioid crisis (Arthur et al. 2023).

When applying safer monitoring and/or opioid prescribing practices as recommended in the CDC guidelines, both clinicians and patients encounter significant barriers. These barriers include: (1) limited access to non-opioid treatments; (2) the urgent pressure for immediate pain relief; (3) patient understanding, expectations, and experiences; (4) prescriber pressures; and (5) reluctance to change (Cross et al. 2022). Both patients and providers often perceive a lack of viable alternatives to opioids for effective pain management, viewing opioids as a necessary last resort. Pain relief is a high priority for patients due to its profound impact on quality of life, and many are willing to accept opioid-related risks in exchange for "adequate" relief. Patients' limited access to clear, consistent information about opioid pain medications further complicates decision-making around opioid use. Providers face challenges, including insufficient training, systemic barriers, and emotional strain when altering pain treatment plans. Implementing alternative pain management strategies is often hampered by high costs, inadequate insurance coverage, limited access in rural areas, and patient-level barriers like financial hardship and transportation. Clinicians may also hesitate to change practices due to concerns about negative outcomes or harm to the patient-provider relationship.

At the same time, prescribers and patients also report four key supports for safer opioid use for pain management, including (1) increased awareness of opioid-related harms and the benefits of deprescribing, (2) clear communication and expectations, (3) support systems for patients, and (4) support for prescribers (Cross et al. 2022). Some patients have initiated discussions about stopping opioids and reported improved functioning, better quality of life, and stable pain levels after discontinuation. Prescribers emphasize the importance of early, ongoing conversations and a shared understanding that deprescribing is gradual and dynamic. Social support from family and friends is essential, as is collaboration among healthcare providers. Prescribers also describe opioid contracts with patients as a supportive tool to help set clear expectations with patients who continue opioid treatment. Other supports for safer pain management include efforts to enhance patients' self-management of their pain, such as improving knowledge and understanding of pain conditions, setting treatment goals, fostering a supportive environment, and ensuring access to a range of treatment options (Spink et al. 2021).

8.2 Introduction to Academic Detailing (AD)

Developed in the 1980s, academic detailing (AD) is traditionally a one-on-one educational outreach intervention to providers and clinicians, centering around implementing evidence-based information and practices on a specific topic (Davis et al. n.d.). Academic detailers engage in one-on-one or small group conversations about a topic, utilizing current evidence-based practices, clinical guidelines, and the latest research to improve patient care and clinical decision-making. It involves trained professionals, often pharmacists, physicians, nurses, or other healthcare experts, visiting clinicians in their workplace, delivering AD education. Educational materials utilize key messages that are tailored to the specific provider's needs and knowledge gaps. The goal of AD is to foster a collaborative dialogue, allowing clinicians to ask questions and engage in discussions that respect their expertise and experiences.

Studies have shown AD to be an effective and feasible educational method in various settings, especially in influencing prescribing behaviors in primary care and enhancing the overall quality of patient care. For example, studies highlighted by the National Resource Center for Academic Detailing, or NaRCAD, demonstrate the positive impact of AD on clinical practice. AD programs have shown success in various domains, including reducing unnecessary antibiotic use and promoting cost-effective medication strategies (Ndefo et al. 2017). Research highlights that one of the key advantages of AD is its ability to foster sustained behavior change in clinicians through a collaborative and non-confrontational approach (Rome et al. 2025). By providing peer-reviewed, evidence-based information in a manner that respects the practitioner's autonomy, AD helps create an opportunity for improvement by fostering a culture of learning rather than one of judgment or punishment.

One notable example of this approach in action is within the Department of Veterans Affairs (VA). The VA has developed a robust and impactful AD program over the past two decades. In 2016, Dr. Gallagher outlined six essential elements (key messages) of effective management for veterans' chronic pain (Gallagher 2016). These elements became central to an evidence-based AD initiative promoted by the VA that integrated the elements into provider and clinician education and support. The six key elements include:

- Educating veterans/families and promote self-efficacy
- Educating and training all team members
- Developing nonpharmacologic modalities
- Instituting safe medication prescribing, including safe opioid use (universal precautions)
- Bringing the veteran's expanded team together through virtual pain consulting, education, and ongoing communication between team members
- Establishing metrics to monitor pain care

While about 30% of the U.S. population experiences chronic pain, the rate is significantly higher within the VA system, especially among older veterans, reaching an estimated 50%. According to Gallagher (2016), this elevated prevalence was driven by the complex physical, psychiatric, and social comorbidities affecting this population, including substance use disorders (SUD), depression, and post-traumatic stress disorder (PTSD), leading to a higher rate of chronic pain.

One of the unique features of clinical pain practice in the VA is the important and growing role of pharmacists with pain management training in the clinical pain team (Gallagher 2016). The Pharmacy Benefits Management Office established AD services at the VA to support the Opioid and Psychotropic Drug Safety Initiatives (U.S. Department of Veterans Affairs, Pharmacy Benefits Management, National Academic Detailing Services 2025). AD creates and provides patient- and provider-level tools designed for AD visits with pain teams and with individual providers needing support while addressing questions related to optimal medications and other treatment modalities. The AD service at the VA also aids in post-training continuing education to providers. Overall, this AD educational method promotes a culture of continuous learning and evidence-driven clinical practice that ultimately helps improve patient safety and outcomes.

8.2.1 *Academic Detailing as a Strategy for Safer Opioid Prescribing*

AD is a tailored, interactive educational outreach intervention that addresses both patient- and provider-level barriers to improve opioid safety and promote effective and evidence-based pain management. Although opioid-related AD interventions have varied in design and evaluated different metrics and outcomes, in general, they have been feasible and effective in terms of changing opioid and naloxone prescribing rates, addressing provider knowledge gaps, and influencing provider adherence to guidelines (Kulbokas et al. 2021; Foster et al. 2023; Kattan et al, 2016; Liebschutz et al. 2017; Williams et al. 2024).

One study examined the variations in implementing AD among 11 of the 29 jurisdictions receiving funding from the CDC to prevent prescription drug overdoses (Underwood et al. 2022). Three AD models were compared and contrasted, including a one-on-one model, train-the-trainer (ToT) model, and a hybrid model. Most programs utilized a one-on-one AD model (nine total) where a trained academic detailer visits a healthcare practice for individual, tailored meetings with providers about how to integrate best practices into their clinical workflows. All nine programs using the one-on-one AD model either tailored or developed a curriculum for AD sessions, which included implementation guides, support webinars, policy papers, and online resources. This tailoring of resources allowed AD teams to target behaviors and outcomes they perceived as most relevant to address opioid overdose in their communities while maintaining fidelity to the principles of AD.

Only one program described in the review utilized the ToT model in addition to the one-on-one AD model (Underwood et al. 2022). The ToT model involves a centrally trained expert educating clinical staff individually or in small groups on how to implement AD. These staff members are then assigned to local areas or organizations to implement AD sessions with clinicians. Similar to one-on-one detailing sessions, the trained expert is responsible for compiling any resources necessary for competence in AD, such as policy papers or online resources (i.e., NaRCAD's opioid overdose implementation guide; NaRCAD n.d.). The primary benefit of the ToT model was that it increased the reach of the intervention by expanding the number of personnel available to conduct AD visits.

Two AD programs reviewed used a hybrid model of clinical training. Although this approach is not typically considered traditional AD, the programs referred to their efforts as such in their reports and qualitative interviews, highlighting group presentations, virtual training, or webinars with clinicians where prescribing guidelines were discussed (Underwood et al. 2022). One example of such group presentations is through Project ECHO, where providers receive personalized feedback and mentoring related to a specific clinical case, such as prescribing medications for opioid use disorder (Morgan et al. 2021). Despite differences between the models, common themes emerged from the Underwood study, including the need to use local data to target AD efforts and the importance of partnerships (Underwood et al. 2022). See Table 8.1 for differences in AD models.

Table 8.1 Comparison of three AD models: one-on-one, train-the-trainer, and hybrid

Feature	*One-on-one academic detailing*	*Train-the-trainer model*	*Hybrid model*
Primary interaction	Direct clinician–detailer interaction	Trainer equips others to detail clinicians	Mix of detailing methods (1:1, group, remote)
Target audience	Individual clinicians	Future academic detailers (e.g., healthcare professionals, peers)	Clinicians and trainers vary by context
Delivery method	In-person, office-based sessions, tailored to the clinician	Workshops, structured training sessions	Combination of in-person, virtual, and group formats
Core goal	Influence clinical decision-making at the point of care	Build workforce capacity for broader dissemination	Flexibility and scalability across diverse settings
Customization level	Highly tailored	Standardized training: Adaptation depends on the trainees	Varies: May include personalized, group, or asynchronous delivery
Follow-up	Follow-up visits often included	May include peer support, check-ins	May include digital or live reinforcement strategies

(*continued*)

Table 8.1 (continued)

Feature	*One-on-one academic detailing*	*Train-the-trainer model*	*Hybrid model*
Scalability	Limited by time and personnel	High: Amplifies reach through new trainers	High: Blends scalable and targeted elements
Examples of use	Evidence-based medication counseling to prescribers	Naloxone education for healthcare professionals who then teach communities	Jurisdictional programs using digital, live, and train-the-trainer methods

While the structure and delivery of AD may differ across models, each approach shares the overarching goal of improving clinical decision-making through evidence-based engagement. Building on these models, targeted AD initiatives have been increasingly tailored to address specific public health challenges, such as the opioid crisis, by integrating tools like the Prescription Drug Monitor Program (PDMP) into clinician outreach and education. These programmatic adaptations demonstrate how AD can evolve to meet emerging needs, offering clinicians both personalized support and actionable resources to enhance prescribing safety.

To help curb overprescribing of opioids, all U.S. states have implemented a PDMP, allowing healthcare providers to track their prescribing patterns (via provider report cards) and compare them with those of their peers in similar specialties (e.g., obstetrics, primary care, geriatrics). In South Carolina, an AD initiative by a clinical pharmacist detailer offered hands-on PDMP training with registration assistance that resulted in a 40.4-fold increase in PDMP utilization compared to pre-AD intervention levels (Ball et al. 2021). The result highlights how targeted AD efforts can directly promote safer prescribing behavior. Rather than simply providing clinical guidelines, AD empowers providers with personalized, evidence-based, and practical tools to navigate complex prescribing decisions. In doing so, it enhances provider confidence and supports more nuanced discussions around pain management and opioid alternatives.

For instance, a study involving 238 physicians found that those who participated in AD sessions significantly reduced their opioid prescribing compared to matched controls (Laur et al. 2025). The physicians reported that AD effectively addressed key barriers to safe pain management, such as limited confidence or challenging, difficult patient interactions, while reinforcing appropriate opioid prescribing and pain management strategies. Similarly, evidence from 11 U.S. states indicates that AD helped reduce variability in opioid prescribing and promoted more judicious prescribing practices across diverse clinical settings, from emergency departments to primary care (Underwood et al. 2022). These studies underscore the efficacy and value of AD in improving opioid prescribing practices while supporting safer, more effective, and evidence-based patient care.

8.3 Launching Effective Academic Detailing Programs

The success of any AD initiative depends not only on its conceptual design but also on its effective implementation. To translate AD's promise into consistent practice change, programs must be grounded in strategic planning and supported by skilled, well-prepared personnel. This section outlines key strategies for implementing impactful AD programs, beginning with guidance on identifying and recruiting the right detailers to lead these efforts.

8.3.1 Recruiting Academic Detailers

There are several important factors to consider when recruiting detailers for an AD program, whether new or established. These factors include a candidate's professional background, communication, writing, facilitation and time management skills, and the time and resources they can dedicate to the program (National Resource Center for Academic Detailing n.d.). Connecting with currently engaged healthcare professionals to gauge their interest in AD roles is a recommended approach. If making new connections, prioritize candidates with strong foundations in relevant fields or professions such as public health, medicine, pharmacy, physical therapy, or nursing. NaRCAD also recommends considering individuals with sales experience, as they often are skilled at navigating resistance or rejection. Additionally, experience or training in motivational interviewing can be highly beneficial because such expertise can encourage "change talk," a technique that elicits a provider's own arguments for behavior change, such as expressing concern about a current prescribing habit or articulating reasons to consider alternatives. For example, during an AD session, a clinician might say, "I've been thinking about the risks of co-prescribing benzodiazepines and opioids," or "I'd like to try a different approach for my patients with chronic pain." These statements reflect an internal motivation for change, which skilled detailers can reinforce using non-confrontational, evidence-based dialogue to evoke and reinforce change talk.

Because the ability to recognize and guide these conversations is closely tied to broader interpersonal strengths, communication skills are another crucial consideration. An ideal candidate will possess excellent interpersonal skills, feel comfortable speaking across disciplines, and be able to facilitate AD sessions that engage clinicians as adult learners. Effective AD requires more than delivering information; it involves encouraging reflection, discussion, and practical application of knowledge. This is where adult learning theories become particularly relevant. For instance, reflective models support the development of reflective practice by encouraging clinicians to examine their current prescribing habits and decision-making processes (Resnicow and McMaster 2012). Constructivism emphasizes learning through experience and action, aligning well with interactive detailing sessions that use real-world patient cases. Transformative learning theory highlights the importance of critical incident analysis and group discussion, which can help clinicians reevaluate underlying assumptions about opioid prescribing and explore new approaches. By drawing on these principles, detailers can better facilitate meaningful, provider-centered conversations that lead to behavior change (Mukhalalati and Taylor 2019). Strong writing and facilitation skills, along with solid time management abilities, are also important for documenting interactions and disseminating key AD messages using program-provided materials. These competencies help ensure that AD efforts are both well-coordinated and effectively communicated across clinical disciplines.

Finally, it is essential to assess the detailer candidate's availability and the resources they can contribute to the AD project. NaRCAD offers immersive and interactive two half-day training sessions for new detailers and encourages participation in regular group check-in webinars to support ongoing skill development. Most detailers dedicate a portion of their time to providing AD interventions on a part-time basis, in addition to their other professional responsibilities, such as teaching, grant initiatives, or patient care. While employing part-time detailers can offer budgetary flexibility, it may also introduce scheduling limitations that impact the ability to deliver services when providers request them. Surveying providers in advance to assess their needs and sharing those requests promptly with detailers on an ad hoc basis can help ensure better scheduling alignment and responsiveness.

8.3.2 *Planning for Detailing Visits*

Before initiating an AD visit with a provider or clinician, it is recommended to first conduct a field test of the educational handouts, commonly referred to as detailing aids. In this context, an academic detailer will pilot the detailing aids in simulated sessions with colleagues, subject matter experts, or a small group of clinicians who are not the primary audience but can provide constructive feedback. These sessions allow detailers to practice delivering key messages in a realistic setting and to assess how clinicians might respond, both verbally and nonverbally, to the content of the detailing aids and delivery style. Feedback from these sessions often yields valuable insights regarding message clarity, tone, length, and clinical relevance. When preparing field testing questions, detailers should consider questions such as: Are the key messages clear and concise? Do they feel actionable? Is the language appropriate for the intended clinical audience? How likely is it for critical concerns or objections to arise? Summary reports of the field testing can be analyzed for common themes, which can then inform revisions to the detailing aid content before full implementation.

To guide the structure of an AD visit, NaRCAD outlines *six key steps* for effective engagement with clinicians (see Fig. 8.1). These include:

1. *Introduction* and rapport-building between the detailer and clinician,
2. *Needs assessment* to understand the clinician's priorities (often in survey forms and through qualitative questions),
3. *Key message* delivery using evidence-based content (via detailing aids),
4. *Addressing objections or barriers* often via a non-confrontational, motivational interviewing approach,
5. *Summarizing key points*, and
6. *Closing the visit* with agreed-upon next steps.

This structured framework guides detailers in creating focused, collaborative conversations that promote behavior change without being prescriptive. While the six-step model provides a foundational structure for conducting AD visits, program teams can further enhance engagement and sustainability by leveraging existing resources and relationships.

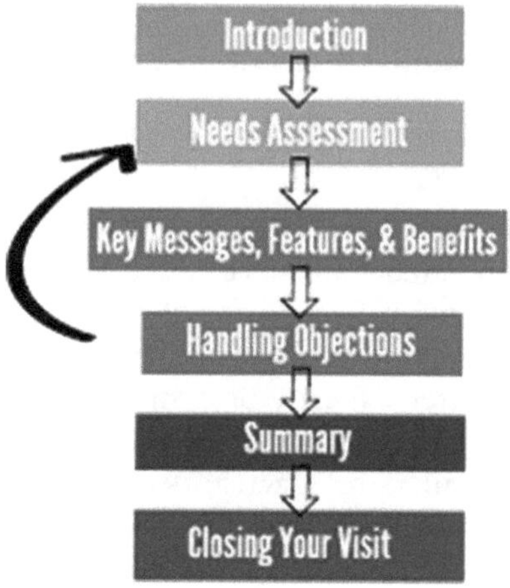
Introduction
Needs Assessment
Key Messages, Features, & Benefits
Handling Objections
Summary
Closing Your Visit

Fig. 8.1 Model to conducting academic detailing visits

Actionable strategies, such as utilizing institutional networks or involving students, can significantly extend the reach and impact of an AD initiative. For example, the AD program at the University of Arkansas for Medical Sciences (UAMS) leveraged its existing partnership with a Federally Qualified Health Center (FQHC)—established through a separate Geriatric Workforce Enhancement Program—to strengthen the participation of FQHC providers in virtual AD sessions on evidence-based chronic pain management, including naloxone prescribing education (Tobey-Moore 2025).

8.3.3 Additional Tips for a Successful AD Visit

When trained detailers meet with a new provider for an AD visit, several important strategies have been discussed in the literature (Soumerai 1990) and by NaRCAD to improve the effectiveness of the interactions. First, the detailer should establish credibility early by being transparent with credentials, mentioning affiliations, and making it clear they are there to support the provider and not "police" or judge practices. It is helpful to understand each specific provider's gaps in knowledge by asking what they currently know about a topic, how they are currently implementing related evidence-based practices, and what challenges they have faced with implementation efforts. When recommending specific changes to a provider's practices, it is helpful to ask them which key messages or actions they feel would be most beneficial for them to implement at this time. By focusing on provider-selected key messages, the detailer will avoid overwhelming the provider with information and improve the likelihood of their successful implementation of the evidence-based practice.

When detailers discuss a topic and key messages with a provider, it is useful to deploy active listening and motivational interviewing techniques (Koh-Knox 2009). Trained detailers should practice these skills before meeting with target providers to improve impact. Examples include reflecting on what the provider tells the detailer, showing empathy and being non-judgmental, and providing guidance and support rather than instruction. Often during these discussions, providers will identify specific barriers and misconceptions that detailers should be prepared to address with up-to-date, evidence-based research. Evidence-based research can include related clinical guidelines, meta-analysis, research trials, and local data. It is helpful to anticipate common questions so detailers can be better prepared with research citations and summaries. If unsure of the answer to provider questions, it is important for the detailer to let the provider know they are "unsure at this time" but will follow up quickly with helpful information. This supports the credibility of the detailer with the provider. Following the detailing session, detailers will often leave educational handouts with providers that include the actionable key messages to encourage clinical practice change, quick summaries of related local and national data, and references for additional evidence-based resources.

Some additional strategies to improve the effectiveness of AD interventions include respecting the provider's time, encouraging collaboration by involving other relevant clinic staff, and incorporating real-life success stories. To increase the likelihood of successfully meeting with providers and delivering key messages, AD meetings should be scheduled in advance and kept brief (10–15 minutes). Keeping visits concise also enhances the provider's ability to retain and apply the information. Framing the relationship as a partnership, such as "We are working together to improve patient outcomes," can foster greater engagement. Pulling in other relevant clinic staff to discuss strategies and possible workflows to implement changes to practice can be beneficial. Sharing examples of how other clinics or providers have implemented similar changes and the positive outcomes they've achieved can serve as powerful motivation. It is also crucial to follow up with providers and offer ongoing support to continue fostering collaborative relationships. Detailers should leave contact information and schedule a specific time with the provider to check back in. To continue the supportive relationship, detailers should continue to share updated resources with providers, including new clinical guidelines, journal articles and tools that have been recently published on the topic of interest.

Tailoring communication to individual providers based on their prescribing patterns and patient populations is essential for effective AD implementation. Many AD programs use statewide data, or health system-based data when applicable, to identify providers who are out of the normal range with opioid prescribing rates. Others take a broader approach, targeting providers in high-risk counties with elevated opioid prescribing and overdose rates. In states like Arkansas, the AD program enhances provider engagement by customizing sessions based on pre-session needs assessments. These conversational assessments help detailers understand the provider's baseline knowledge, attitudes toward the CDC pain management guidelines, current naloxone co-prescribing practices, and perceptions of local opioid dispensing trends as compared to national trends (Tobey-Moore et al. 2025). This individualized assessment encourages providers to share their specific experiences and concerns, allowing the detailer to tailor key messages and information to their learning needs and clinical context. It is important to end detailing sessions with a summary of the key messages or follow up actions the provider can take, and a gentle ask for a commitment to specific changes in practice, such as improving co-prescribing of naloxone with opioids, in alignment with evidence-based guidelines and research (Tobey-Moore et al. 2025).

8.4 Building an Impactful Academic Detailing Program

Every AD visit is an opportunity to build trust, tailor messages to the provider's unique needs, and reinforce key points that encourage sustainable practice change. However, the success of AD visits hinges greatly on the effectiveness of an AD program. This section outlines several strategies, including creating robust evaluation plans, crafting impactful detailing aids, and engaging learners in the initiatives, that can be adopted to build an impactful AD program.

8.4.1 Planning for Evaluation

Whether or not an AD program is linked to a formal research study, evaluation is essential for understanding its effectiveness and ensuring long-term sustainability. The first step in this process is identifying the specific data the program aims to collect. This involves determining which outcomes align with the AD program's goals, such as changes in prescribing behavior, increased provider confidence, or improved knowledge, and ensuring that the necessary data is both accessible and of sufficient quality. Not all meaningful outcomes can be easily quantified, so it's important to clearly define the purpose of the assessment and the intended audience of the assessment report, whether stakeholders, funders, or internal quality improvement teams.

Once those considerations are addressed, the program team can begin to visualize what kinds of outputs they hope to produce, such as summary tables, figures, or narrative reports. These outputs should be grounded in clear, purposeful evaluation questions. For instance, are providers more confident in prescribing naloxone after the AD visit? Have they gained a stronger understanding of non-opioid options for managing chronic pain? Do their prescribing patterns reflect increased alignment with evidence-based guidelines? These types of questions help guide evaluation efforts and ensure that the data collected is actionable.

Data may be either quantitative or qualitative, or ideally, both. Quantitative data might include the number of AD visits completed, changes in opioid prescribing behavior sourced from PDMPs, or pre/post survey scores reflecting changes in provider knowledge, competence, or confidence. Qualitative data could include provider comments, quotes, or reflections on barriers and motivators for behavior change. Observations made during AD sessions, particularly regarding provider engagement, hesitations, or even resistance, can also provide powerful context information.

Data may also be collected from various sources, including local or state health departments, insurance claims data, CDC dashboards, provider surveys, and internal AD program tracking tools. The program team should first consider free or existing datasets, if available, before initiating large-scale needs assessments that may be resource- and cost-intensive. In some cases, such as in Arkansas, provider-level opioid prescribing data may be inaccessible outside specific healthcare systems like the United States

Department of Veterans Affairs (VA), so anticipating and planning for such limitations is important.

AD programs also need to select appropriate tools for data collection and management. Platforms such as REDCap, Qualtrics, Salesforce, SurveyMonkey, Google Forms, or Microsoft Forms can be used depending on institutional access, data security needs, and staff familiarity. These tools can help track both process metrics and outcomes over time. To measure the impact of AD interventions, it's advisable to collect data at multiple time points. Programs might conduct surveys or assessments before AD visits, immediately following a detailing visit, then at longitudinal intervals such as 1–2 weeks, 30 days, or 90 days post-AD visit. The frequency and timing of these assessments should be guided by the nature of the intervention and the outcomes being measured.

The overarching goal is to thoughtfully consider and systematically collect data that speaks to the AD program's intended impact. This ensures that short-term quality improvement needs are addressed while also building a foundation for long-term program sustainability and potential replication. At minimum, the detailer will want to capture provider demographic data and AD visit data (see Fig. 8.2).

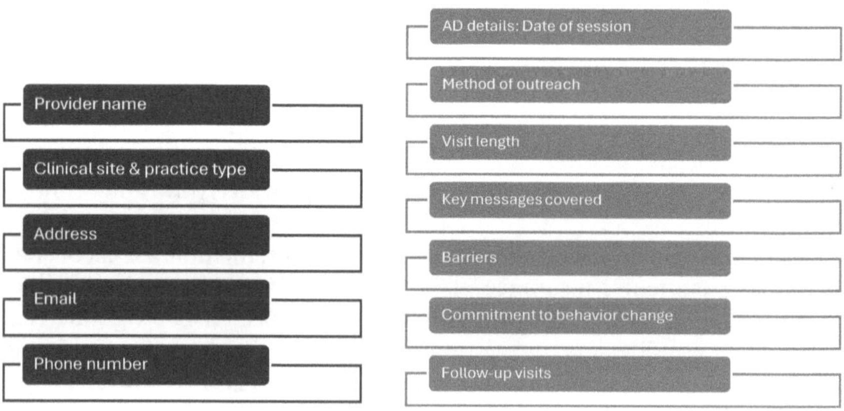

Fig. 8.2 Provider demographic data and AD visit data

8.4.2 Creating and Implementing Impactful Detailing Aids

Beyond measuring outcomes through robust data collection, ensuring the success of AD efforts also requires delivering content in a format that is clear, concise, and actionable for providers. Well-crafted detailing aids (e.g., educational brochure or handout) help distill complex clinical information into specific key messages that are memorable and implement-ready. These concise, often one-page (front and back), documents serve as visual guides during the AD visits and provide a structure that allows the detailer to personalize messaging to each provider's needs, priorities, obstacles, and clinical setting. According to NaRCAD, several principles are necessary to designing impactful detailing aids.

- *Simplify* complex clinical evidence through clear visuals and easy-to-understand graphics.
- *Emphasize* key messages that align with specific, desired clinical behavior changes.
- *Incorporate* elements that engage multiple learning styles to encourage interaction and discussion.
- *Include* tangible, actionable resources that clinicians can reference after the session.

When tied directly to the AD Program's goals—whether to improve naloxone prescribing rates, reduce opioid prescribing and dosages, or recommend nonpharmacologic pain therapies—detailing aids become more than just informational handouts. They catalyze clinical behavior change and are a springboard for ongoing provider engagement.

The following is an example of how a detailer might deliver Key Message 1 from a detailing aid shown in Fig. 8.3. The detailer would begin by presenting one to two supporting resources, such as the CDC's 2022 Clinical Practice Guidelines for Prescribing Opioids for Pain, which emphasize that pain reduction (not complete elimination) is the primary goal of pain care and treatment. To bring this message to life, the detailer could introduce a case-based scenario: for instance, a 35-year-old male patient who sustained a partial-thickness, second-degree burn to his hand and wrist during a kitchen grease fire. The patient endorses experiencing intense pain during dressing changes, interfering with sleep and daily function. In this context, a short-term prescription of a low-dose opioid (e.g., 5 mg hydrocodone for 2–3 days) may be warranted to facilitate healing and

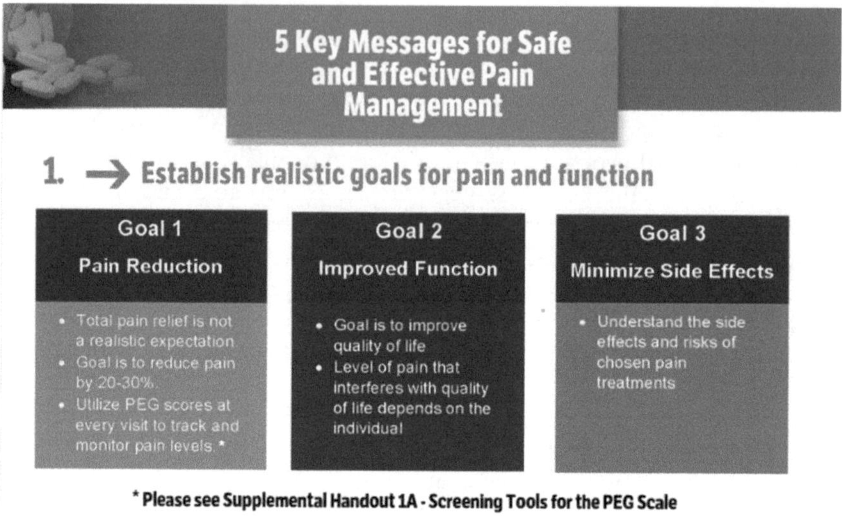

Fig. 8.3 Example of academic detailing key messages

improve short-term function. This scenario allows the detailer to emphasize realistic pain goals, such as aiming for a 20–30% reduction in pain, improving daily activities, and minimizing treatment side effects, consistent with the goals listed in the detailing aid (see Fig. 8.3).

Next, after delivering the key message, the AD session might proceed with an actionable item, often framed as a motivational interviewing question. For example, the detailer might ask the clinician: "How do you currently communicate the short-term nature of opioid use to your patients, emphasizing the risk of dependence and need for naloxone when necessary?" This format encourages reflection on the practitioner's current practices while emphasizing the importance of patient safety and timely follow-up. Then, the detailer might share the second key message on the AD materials with the provider.

Generally speaking, when designing detailing aids, five elements—clinic problem, evidence snapshot, key messages, provider action items, and resources—should be considered to ensure the content is both clinically relevant and strategically organized. These elements help frame the clinical issue, reinforce evidence-based guidance, and provide practical tools that support provider behavior change during AD sessions. Each element plays a specific role in guiding the conversation, reinforcing key messages, and prompting providers to take actionable steps aligned with best practices. Here is an example of a detailing aid outline including all five elements.

1. **Clinical Problem (Top Section)**

   - Brief statement on local or regional data related to prescribing and using opioids (e.g., prescribing trends, overdose data).
   - Local, state, and national data snapshots frame the importance of the issue.

2. **Evidence Snapshot**

   - Summary of key CDC guidelines or other evidence-based clinical recommendations.
   - Relevant local data (e.g., PDMP trends, naloxone prescribing rates).
   - One brief, evidence-based rationale or case for intervention.

3. **Key Messages (Central Section)**

   - Prioritize non-opioid therapies for chronic pain management.
   - If opioids are necessary, start with the lowest effective dose and shortest duration.
   - Always assess risk and consider co-prescribing naloxone for at-risk patients.
   - Use shared decision-making and taper when appropriate.
   - An example of an academic detailer's approach to evidence-based pain management might begin with one to three key messages, see Fig. 8.3 for an example of one key message.

4. **Provider Action Items**

   - Identify one or more patients for tapering discussion.
   - Co-prescribe naloxone for patients at risk of accidental overdose.
   - Initiative or refer for non-opioid therapies (e.g., physical therapy, Cognitive Behavioral Therapy [CBT], topical analgesics).
   - Review PDMP and document risk assessment along with naloxone education in the Electronic Medical Records (EMR).

5. **Resources (Bottom Section)**

- Links to local naloxone laws or standing orders.
- Links to and phone numbers of local harm reduction organizations that may provide free naloxone kits directly to patients.
- Quick reference to opioid tapering protocol.
- Printable or digital patient education handouts.
- Contact information for AD program support or follow-up.

8.4.3 Engagement of Learners in Initiatives

Engaging students in AD initiatives, particularly students in the fields of pharmacy, medicine, physical therapy, nursing, or public health, can serve as both a workforce development strategy and a means of enriching the initiatives. UAMS launched a multidisciplinary AD program in 2021 and expanded its efforts by offering a research-focused AD fellowship opportunity to pharmacy students in 2023. A second-year PharmD student trained using publicly available materials provided by NaRCAD not only participated in live detailing sessions but also contributed to the development of tailored educational materials and detailing aids, adding capacity and innovation to the program. Beyond programmatic contributions, early educational exposure to AD principles helps students internalize core clinical communication skills. For example, a combined training initiative described in the literature integrated naloxone-focused AD with hands-on naloxone administration in a pharmacy skills lab (Evoy et al. 2020; Kavanaugh et al. 2021). This model allowed students to practice both evidence-based outreach and clinical intervention under statewide standing orders, reinforcing the value of unbiased communication, patient-centered care, and the translation of public health strategies into practice. AD thus represents a valuable and underutilized avenue for experiential learning that prepares students to apply population health tools such as naloxone education more confidently in their future careers.

8.5 Case Studies of AD Initiatives

To further illustrate the application of AD in opioid-related clinical contexts, we highlight ten case studies that demonstrate how AD has been implemented to address different aspects of opioid safety. In each example, we describe how the authors structured their detailing interventions, the challenges encountered, and the observed outcomes. Collectively, these case studies reflect the adaptability of AD across settings, from national health systems to local pharmacies, and offer insights into how provider education can be tailored to improve clinical practices related to opioid prescribing, naloxone access, and the use of tools such as PDMPs.

8.5.1 Case 1: Evidence-Based Interventions to Improve Opioid Prescribing in Primary Care: A Qualitative Assessment of Implementation in Two Studies

Caroll and colleagues examined the randomized controlled trials conducted at TOPCARE (Opioid Therapy in Primary Care) and TEACH (Targeting Effective Approaches to Chronic HIV Care) that tested an intervention designed to promote guideline-adherent long-term opioid therapy (LTOT; Carroll et al. 2023). The intervention combined AD, a nurse care manager, and an electronic registry to support safer prescribing. Providers viewed the intervention positively, but challenges with workflow integration and long-term sustainability emerged. This case underscores the importance of relationship-building and system-level support in sustaining AD efforts.

8.5.2 Case 2: Improving the Delivery of Chronic Opioid Therapy Among People Living with Human Immunodeficiency Virus: A Cluster-Randomized Clinical Trial

This unblinded, cluster-randomized trial evaluated the TEACH intervention—AD delivered by nurse care managers with electronic registry support and addiction specialist access—among healthcare providers treating patients living with HIV who are prescribed chronic opioid therapy (COT; Samet et al. 2021). Compared to providers who did not receive the AD intervention, those receiving it were significantly more likely to adhere to COT guidelines, including higher rates of urine drug testing (71% vs. 20%; $p < 0.0001$). The study showed that team-based care with dedicated nurse support can enhance safe prescribing without increasing provider burden.

8.5.3 Case 3: Providers' Perceptions on Barriers and Facilitators to Prescribing Naloxone for Patients at Risk for Opioid Overdose After Implementation of a National AD Program: A Qualitative Assessment

In this national VA study, AD interventions were used to encourage naloxone prescribing among providers caring for veterans at risk of overdose (Bounthavong et al. 2020). Providers appreciated the AD model but cited barriers to implementing the recommended practice such as stigma, limited resources for vulnerable populations, and poor data integration. Besides barriers, they also mentioned factors facilitating the implementation of the practice, including follow-up AD visits and personalized virtual sessions. This case highlights the value of contextualizing AD to address structural and social barriers.

8.5.4 Case 4: Impact of Implementing an AD Program on Opioid-Benzodiazepine Co-Prescribing Trends at the U.S. Department of Veterans Affairs

This follow-up VA study to Bounthavong et al. (2020) evaluated the impact of AD on high-risk opioid-benzodiazepine co-prescribing trends (Bounthavong et al. 2021). Implemented across 119 VA sites, the intervention led to a 33% greater reduction in co-prescribing at sites with AD exposure. The finding demonstrates the dose-response impact of AD: greater provider exposure led to greater improvements, emphasizing the benefits of broad implementation of AD within large systems.

8.5.5 Case 5: AD Increases Prescription Drug Monitoring Program Use Among Primary Care Practices

In a statewide initiative, Ball and colleagues deployed AD to increase PDMP use in primary care (Ball et al. 2021). A clinical pharmacist delivered training and hands-on support to prescribers and PDMP delegates; these delegates were nurses or medical assistants authorized by the prescribers to query the state's PDMP on their behalf. Following the intervention, PDMP report requests, especially by delegates, rose dramatically. This case illustrates how AD can drive immediate changes in clinical behavior.

8.5.6 Case 6: Impact of Student Pharmacist-Led Naloxone AD at Community Pharmacies in Texas

Evoy and colleagues piloted a student-led AD initiative in Texas community pharmacies to improve naloxone accessibility (Evoy et al. 2020). After conducting telephone audits, student pharmacists visited pharmacies to deliver brief, targeted education on standing orders and overdose response. Naloxone stocking, dispensing to third parties, and insurance claims all increased post-intervention. This case showcases the scalability and promise of engaging student detailers to expand naloxone access.

8.5.7 Case 7: Combining Simulated AD with Naloxone Training to Prepare Student Pharmacists for Opioid Risk Mitigation Strategies

Kavanaugh and her colleagues reported a unique educational activity integrating AD and hands-on naloxone training for student pharmacists in an accelerated pharmacy program (Kavanaugh et al. 2021). Incorporating AD into naloxone training allowed students to gain skills of assessing the needs of patients and providers and addressing concerns using evidence-based communication. The authors noted that no other pharmacy programs had combined AD with naloxone training and contended that this approach may help shift societal perceptions and improve naloxone access. Key lessons learned included the value of early AD exposure, involving non-student volunteers for realistic practice, using varied learning techniques, and enhancing feedback. The model offers a promising way to strengthen real-world communication skills and could benefit from mixed-methods evaluation.

8.5.8 Case 8: AD for Postpartum Opioid Prescribing

This quality improvement project aimed to improve opioid prescribing for postpartum women at one medical center (Voelker and Schauberger 2018). Nineteen prescribers received baseline prescribing data and AD intervention. Following the intervention, median opioid tablets per prescription dropped by five, and average MME decreased from 171 to 143 ($p = 0.001$). Post-cesarean opioid prescribing declined from 100% to 93% ($p = 0.054$), with a significant reduction in tablet count ($p = 0.0002$). For vaginal deliveries, prescribing fell from 15% to 9% ($p = 0.03$), with no significant change in tablet count. Lessons learned included recognizing the underused potential of data from the electronic health record in such projects and considering the influence of concurrent tools like PDMPs. The study highlights the value of provider-level prescribing data in assessing AD impact and suggests future work could link patient outcomes to specific prescribers to better assess effectiveness.

8.5.9 *Case 9: The Feasibility of AD for Acute and Oral Pain Management in Outpatient Dentistry: A Pilot Study*

This pilot study explored the feasibility of an AD intervention to promote guideline-based opioid prescribing for acute oral pain in outpatient dentistry (Hughes et al. 2023). Five dentists at a Midwestern VA dental clinic received one-on-one AD sessions from a pharmacy-trained pain management detailer, along with a one-page guideline handout. Most dentists were receptive to the intervention and viewed the detailer as engaged and responsive. A difference-in-difference analysis showed a downward trend in opioid prescribing among participating dentists. Key lessons learned included the value of pairing education with tailored support materials and offering individualized feedback. The study highlights AD's adaptability across clinical settings and emphasizes the importance of assessing feasibility before wider implementation.

8.5.10 *Case 10: Feasibility and Acceptability of Virtual AD on Opioid Prescribing*

This study examined the feasibility and acceptability of virtual AD on appropriate opioid prescribing during the COVID-19 pandemic when social distancing was required (Smart et al. 2021). An initial in-person AD visit was followed by a virtual visit within eight weeks. Videoconferencing was the primary method of communication, with the telephone as a backup. Virtual visits had slightly lower completion rates compared to in-person visits (77% vs. 90%), and provider satisfaction scores were slightly lower for virtual visits (mean difference = -2.94, $p < 0.001$). There was no significant difference in detailer perceptions between visit types. Future research should evaluate the impact of different visit modalities on outcomes such as prescribing behaviors.

8.6 Conclusion

For future improvement, AD programs should focus on strengthening evaluation strategies, improving program efficiency, and advancing targeted research. Key priorities include developing standardized metrics to measure impact, fostering collaboration across programs, and generating evidence to support sustainable, cost-effective implementation—while continuing to improve communication with healthcare providers and the overall impact of interventions. As demonstrated in a recent systematic review, standardized evaluation metrics, such as provider adherence to evidence-based guideline recommendations, are essential for assessing the effectiveness of diverse programs (Rome et al. 2025). Establishing a shared set of indicators would enable meaningful comparisons and foster the identification of best practices. Likewise, collaboration between AD programs through a central networking repository would help identify the most effective educational tools and improve program quality and reach. Creating a centralized repository for academic detailers and their resource materials would promote consistency, reduce redundancy, potentially increase productivity, and support more cohesive educational efforts (Rome et al. 2025).

While studies frequently assess short-term outcomes, the long-term sustainability of AD interventions remains unclear and should be a priority for future research. A scoping review of AD interventions related to opioid outcomes highlighted the need for studies that evaluate the durability of behavior change over time (Kulbokas et al. 2021). Comparative effectiveness research is also warranted to determine whether AD is more impactful when used alone or in combination with other strategies, such as audit and feedback. Additional research should explore AD's performance across varied clinical settings and patient populations, the effects of AD on relevant outcomes, such as reductions in inappropriate opioid prescribing, increased naloxone co-prescribing, improved use of non-opioid pain management strategies, and enhanced adherence to clinical guidelines. Finally, cost-effectiveness studies and robust evaluations of AD facilitator training models will be vital in supporting policy decisions by providing lawmakers and health system leaders with evidence on which strategies may have the greatest impact for the investment, which can guide funding allocations, reimbursement models, and public health priorities. By continuing studying and bettering AD, researchers and healthcare practitioners can help shape the future of AD as a dynamic and responsive tool for improving clinical practice and patient outcomes (Kulbokas et al. 2021; Rome et al. 2025).

References

Arthur, Joseph, Tonya Edwards, Zhanni Lu, et al. 2023. Healthcare Provider Perceptions and Reported Practices Regarding Opioid Prescription for Patients with Chronic Pain. *Research Square*, September 27, rs.3.rs-3367358. https://doi.org/10.21203/rs.3.rs-3367358/v1.

Ball, Sarah J., Jenna A. McCauley, Megan Pruitt, et al. 2021. Academic Detailing Increases Prescription Drug Monitoring Program Use among Primary Care Practices. *Journal of the American Pharmacists Association* 61 (4): 418.e2–424.e2. https://doi.org/10.1016/j.japh.2021.02.019.

Bounthavong, Mark, Kangho Suh, Melissa L. D. Christopher, David L. Veenstra, Anirban Basu, and Emily Beth Devine. 2020. Providers' Perceptions on Barriers and Facilitators to Prescribing Naloxone for Patients at Risk for Opioid Overdose after Implementation of a National Academic Detailing Program: A Qualitative Assessment. *Research in Social & Administrative Pharmacy: RSAP* 16 (8): 1033–1040. https://doi.org/10.1016/j.sapharm.2019.10.015.

Bounthavong, Mark, Marcos K. Lau, Chad L. Kay, et al. 2021. Impact of Implementing an Academic Detailing Program on Opioid-Benzodiazepine Co-Prescribing Trends at the U.S. Department of Veterans Affairs. *Pain Medicine* 22 (6): 1426–1434. https://doi.org/10.1093/pm/pnaa475.

Carroll, Jennifer J., Phoebe A. Cushman, Marlene C. Lira, et al. 2023. "Evidence-Based Interventions to Improve Opioid Prescribing in Primary Care: A Qualitative Assessment of Implementation in Two Studies." Journal of General Internal Medicine (United States) 38 (8): 1794–801. https://doi.org/10.1007/s11606-022-07909-3./pp/p.

Centers for Disease Control and Prevention. 2025. *Understanding the Opioid Overdose Epidemic. Overdose Prevention.* July 12. https://www.cdc.gov/overdose-prevention/about/understanding-the-opioid-overdose-epidemic.html.

Cross, Amanda J., Rachelle Buchbinder, Stephanie Mathieson, et al. 2022. Barriers and Enablers to Monitoring and Deprescribing Opioid Analgesics for Chronic Non-Cancer Pain: A Systematic Review with Qualitative Evidence Synthesis Using the Theoretical Domains Framework. *BMJ Quality & Safety* 31 (5): 387–400. https://doi.org/10.1136/bmjqs-2021-014186.

Davis, Margot Trotter, Brian Bateman, and Jerry Avorn. n.d. Educational Outreach to Opioid Prescribers: The Case for Academic Detailing. *Pain Physician* 2017:6.

Dowell, Deborah, Tamara M. Haegerich, and Roger Chou. 2016. CDC Guideline for Prescribing Opioids for Chronic Pain—United States, 2016. *MMWR. Recommendations and Reports: Morbidity and Mortality Weekly Report. Recommendations and Reports* 65 (1): 1–49. https://doi.org/10.15585/mmwr.rr6501e1.

Dowell, Deborah, Kathleen R. Ragan, Christopher M. Jones, Grant T. Baldwin, and Roger Chou. 2022. Prescribing Opioids for Pain—The New CDC Clinical Practice Guideline. *New England Journal of Medicine* 387 (22): 2011–2013. https://doi.org/10.1056/NEJMp2211040.

Evoy, Kirk E., Lindsey Groff, Lucas G. Hill, William Godinez, Ravi Gandhi, and Kelly R. Reveles. 2020. Impact of Student Pharmacist-Led Naloxone Academic Detailing at Community Pharmacies in Texas. *Journal of the American Pharmacists Association: JAPhA* 60 (1): 81–86. https://doi.org/10.1016/j.japh.2019.09.007.

Foster, Carla L., Ellenie Tuazon, Emily Winkelstein, Hillary V. Kunins, and Jessica A. Kattan. 2023. Public Health Detailing to Increase Naloxone Access in NYC Pharmacies. *Journal of the American Pharmacists Association: JAPhA* 63 (3): 885–892. https://doi.org/10.1016/j.japh.2023.03.001.

Gallagher, Rollin M. 2016. Advancing the Pain Agenda in the Veteran Population. *Anesthesiology Clinics* 34 (2): 357–378. https://doi.org/10.1016/j.anclin.2016.01.003.

Hughes, Ashley M., Erica Lin, Raza A. Hussain, et al. 2023. The Feasibility of Academic Detailing for Acute Oral Pain Management in Outpatient Dentistry: A Pilot Study. *Journal of the American Pharmacists Association: JAPhA* 63 (1): 158.e6–163.e6. https://doi.org/10.1016/j.japh.2022.08.001.

Kattan, Jessica A., Ellenie Tuazon, Denise Paone, et al. 2016. Public Health Detailing-A Successful Strategy to Promote Judicious Opioid Analgesic Prescribing. *American Journal of Public Health* 106 (8): 1430–1438. https://doi.org/10.2105/AJPH.2016.303274.

Kavanaugh, Rachel, Mc Kenzie Yerks, Ryan Feldman, and Matthew Stanton. 2021. Combining Simulated Academic Detailing with Naloxone Training to Prepare Student Pharmacists for Opioid Risk Mitigation Strategies. *Currents in Pharmacy Teaching & Learning* 13 (12): 1679–1682. https://doi.org/10.1016/j.cptl.2021.09.030.

Koh-Knox, Cynthia P. 2009. Motivational Interviewing in Health Care: Helping Patients Change Behavior. *American Journal of Pharmaceutical Education* 73 (7): 127.

Kulbokas, Victoria, Kent A. Hanson, Mary H. Smart, Monika Rao Mandava, Todd A. Lee, and A. Simon Pickard. 2021. Academic Detailing Interventions for Opioid-Related Outcomes: A Scoping Review. *Drugs in Context* 10. https://doi.org/10.7573/dic.2021-7-7.

Laur, Celia, Natasha Kithulegoda, Nicola McCleary, et al. 2025. Changing or Validating Physician Opioid Prescribing Behaviors through Audit and Feedback and Academic Detailing Interventions in Primary Care. *Implementation Research and Practice* 6:26334895241307638. https://doi.org/10.1177/26334895241307638.

Liebschutz, Jane M., Ziming Xuan, Christopher W. Shanahan, et al. 2017. Improving Adherence to Long-Term Opioid Therapy Guidelines to Reduce Opioid Misuse in Primary Care: A Cluster-Randomized Clinical Trial. *JAMA Internal Medicine* 177 (9): 1265–1272. https://doi.org/10.1001/jamainternmed.2017.2468.

Morgan, Anna R., Michelle A. Hendricks, Sanae El Ibrahimi, et al. 2021. COVID-19-Related Adaptations to the Implementation and Evaluation of a Clinic-Based Intervention Designed to Improve Opioid Safety. *Drugs in Context* 10. https://doi.org/10.7573/dic.2021-7-5.

Mukhalalati, Banan Abdulrzaq, and Andrea Taylor. 2019. Adult Learning Theories in Context: A Quick Guide for Healthcare Professional Educators. *Journal of Medical Education and Curricular Development* 6:2382120519840332. https://doi.org/10.1177/2382120519840332.

NARCAD. n.d. National Resource Center for Academic Detailing. https://www.narcad.org/. Accessed 9 April 2025.

National Resource Center for Academic Detailing. n.d. AD How-To Guides. NARCAD. https://www.narcad.org/ad-how-to-guides.html. Accessed 18 August 2025.

Ndefo, Uche Anadu, Rolicia Norman, and Andrea Henry. 2017. *Academic Detailing Has a Positive Effect on Prescribing and Decreasing Prescription Drug Costs: A Health Plan's Perspective*. May 16. https://www.ahdbonline.com/issues/2017/may-2017-vol-10-no-3/2369-academic-detailing-has-a-positive-effect-on-prescribing-and-decreasing-prescription-drug-costs-a-health-plan-s-perspective?utm_source=chatgpt.com.

Resnicow, Ken, and Fiona McMaster. 2012. Motivational Interviewing: Moving from Why to How with Autonomy Support. *International Journal of Behavioral Nutrition and Physical Activity* 9 (1): 19. https://doi.org/10.1186/1479-5868-9-19.

Rome, Benjamin N., Ellen Dancel, Alexander Chaitoff, et al. 2025. Academic Detailing Interventions and Evidence-Based Prescribing: A Systematic Review. *JAMA Network Open* 8 (1): e2453684. https://doi.org/10.1001/jamanetworkopen.2024.53684.

Samet, Jeffrey H., Judith I. Tsui, Debbie M. Cheng, et al. 2021. Improving the Delivery of Chronic Opioid Therapy Among People Living With Human Immunodeficiency Virus: A Cluster Randomized Clinical Trial. *Clinical Infectious Diseases* 73 (7): e2052–e2058. https://doi.org/10.1093/cid/ciaa1025.

Smart, Mary H., Monika Rao Mandava, Todd A. Lee, and A. Simon Pickard. 2021. Feasibility and Acceptability of Virtual Academic Detailing on Opioid

Prescribing. *International Journal of Medical Informatics* 147:104365. https://doi.org/10.1016/j.ijmedinf.2020.104365.

Soumerai, Stephen B. 1990. Principles of Educational Outreach ('Academic Detailing') to Improve Clinical Decision Making. *JAMA: The Journal of the American Medical Association* 263 (4): 549. https://doi.org/10.1001/jama.1990.03440040088034.

Spink, Alison, Ilona Wagner, and Paul Orrock. 2021. Common Reported Barriers and Facilitators for Self-Management in Adults with Chronic Musculoskeletal Pain: A Systematic Review of Qualitative Studies. *Musculoskeletal Science & Practice* 56:102433. https://doi.org/10.1016/j.msksp.2021.102433.

Substance Abuse and Mental Health Services Administration. 2024. *Key Substance Use and Mental Health Indicators in the United States: Results from the 2023 National Survey on Drug Use and Health*. HHS Publication No. PEP24-07-021, NSDUH Series H-59. Center for Behavioral Health Statistics and Quality, Substance Abuse and Mental Health Services Administration. https://www.samhsa.gov/data/report/2023-nsduh-annual-national-report.

Tobey-Moore L, Breckling MN, Ali M, Karr M, Massey S, Hudson TJ. 2025. Academic Detailing to Advance Naloxone Prescribing in Rural Primary Care: A 2-Year Pilot Study. J Prim Care Community Health. 2025 Jan-Dec; 16:21501319251391284. https://doi.org/10.1177/21501319251391284. Epub 2025 Nov 12. PMID: 41221541; PMCID: PMC12612510.

U.S. Department of Veterans Affairs, Pharmacy Benefits Management, National Academic Detailing Services. 2025. *Academic Detailing Services—Educational Materials—Pharmacy Benefits Management Services*. July 15. https://www.pbm.va.gov/pbm/academicdetailingservicehome.asp.

U.S. Food and Drug Administration. 2019. *FDA Identifies Harm Reported from Sudden Discontinuation of Opioid Pain Medicines and Requires Label Changes to Guide Prescribers on Gradual, Individualized Tapering*. FDA, December. https://www.fda.gov/drugs/drug-safety-and-availability/fda-identifies-harm-reported-sudden-discontinuation-opioid-pain-medicines-and-requires-label-changes.

U.S. Food and Drug Administration. 2020. *Report to Congress on Opioid Prescribing Limits*. https://www.fda.gov/media/147152/download?utm_source=chatgpt.com.

Underwood, Natasha L., Jessica Duncan Cance, Heather Kane, Caitlin Hennessy, Aleta Christensen, and Cherie Rooks-Peck. 2022. Understanding State-Level Variations in Implementing Academic Detailing for Prescribing Opioids: Findings from 11 States Within the United States. *Pain Medicine* 23 (10): 1644–1653. https://doi.org/10.1093/pm/pnac039.

Voelker, Katya Alcaraz, and Charles Schauberger. 2018. Academic Detailing for Postpartum Opioid Prescribing. *Journal of the American Board of Family*

Medicine: JABFM (United States) 31 (6): 944–946. https://doi.org/10.3122/jabfm.2018.06.180071.

Williams, Emily C., Madeline C. Frost, Mark Bounthavong, et al. 2024. Implementation of Opioid Safety Efforts: Influence of Academic Detailing on Adverse Outcomes Among Patients in the Veterans Health Administration. *Substance Use & Addiction Journal* (United States), 29767342241243309. https://doi.org/10.1177/29767342241243309.

PART III

Communication, Treatment, and Social Support

CHAPTER 9

The Role of Patient-Centered Communication and Navigation in Addressing Barriers to Opioid Use Disorder Treatment Within an Ecological Framework

Jessica Beckham Houck

9.1 Introduction

Imagine the entire population of Charleston, South Carolina, or Boulder, Colorado, being wiped off the map. Or picture the entire student body of Texas A&M, Ohio State University, or the University of Central Florida was suddenly eliminated. Such cataclysmic events would elicit every resource of our state and federal government and command the attention of the entire world. However, would people notice the extent of this same loss if it was spread across the United States over the period of a year? An unyielding plague of opioid deaths largely flies under the radar year after year with little public regard. Since 2021, over 100,000 preventable deaths

J. B. Houck (✉)
Department of Mass Media and Strategic Communication, University of Tennessee at Martin, Martin, TN, USA
e-mail: Jbeckha4@utm.edu

X. Cao (ed.), *Fighting the Opioid Crisis with Communication*,
https://doi.org/10.1007/978-3-032-31162-7_9

have occurred annually due to opioid overdoses (Centers for Disease Control and Prevention [CDC] 2024). These numbers are not merely statistics; they represent lives cut short and families torn apart. Communities are left grappling with the long-term fallout of opioid addiction and are desperately searching for solutions.

That said, recent data suggests encouraging progress, evidenced by a 10% decline in national overdose deaths between April 2023 and April 2024 (CDC 2025a). Opioid overdose victims stand a much better chance at survival today because Emergency Medical Services (EMS) responders, including early responders from the police and fire departments, routinely carry and are trained in the use of naloxone, a medication that can reverse respiratory depression caused by an opioid overdose (Lynn and Galinkin 2018). A field study completed by the New York State Department of Health in conjunction with the New York State Police reviewed 354 naloxone administration reports and found a 99% survival rate (Payne et al. 2024). However, provisional data from the CDC's National Center for Health Statistics highlights that drug-related deaths remain alarmingly high. Experts warn that early decreases in overdose deaths may not yet signal a definitive turning point: this crisis is far from over (CDC 2025a). Naloxone is reducing mortality rates and providing a second chance at life for opioid overdose victims, but without effective systemic support, it is often buying time rather than solving the deeper issues.

The persistence of opioid misuse underscores the urgent need for sustained, multifaceted interventions. Laws and punitive threats do little to dissuade those in the throes of addiction. The opioid epidemic is not merely a crisis of substance use—it is a crisis fueled by inadequate communication, limited healthcare access, and systemic failures across multiple sectors (Substance Abuse and Mental Health Services Administration and Office of the Surgeon General 2016; Volkow et al. 2019). With record opioid settlement funds available to support such efforts (National Academy for State Health Policy 2023), addressing this crisis requires an integrated, public health-oriented strategy that focuses on prevention, treatment, harm reduction, and mitigating stigma.

Central to this approach are two key strategies: patient-centered communication (PCC) and patient navigation. PCC emphasizes empathy, trust-building, shared decision-making, and clear information exchange between providers and patients (Epstein and Street 2007). It can be particularly effective for individuals with opioid use disorder (OUD), who often face stigma, emotional distress, and fragmented healthcare systems

(Bielenberg et al. 2021; McCurry et al. 2023). Complementing PCC, patient navigation provides hands-on assistance with logistical challenges (e.g., accessing treatment, insurance and financial counseling, and securing transportation), helping to ensure that patients follow through on care plans (Freeman 2004; Anvari et al. 2022). Together, these strategies offer practical ways of addressing barriers to OUD care and improving long-term recovery outcomes.

Before these strategies can be effectively deployed, it is essential to examine the complex, overlapping barriers that shape the treatment journey of individuals with OUD. The ecological model of health behavior provides a useful approach to understand how these challenges emerge at different levels—ranging from individual struggles to broader social, organizational, and policy-related barriers. This chapter uses the ecological model to explore these barriers and examines how PCC and patient navigation can help address the barriers and pave the bridge to recovery.

9.2 Barriers to Treatment Across Ecological Levels

The ecological model of health behavior, developed by McLeroy, Bibeau, Steckler, and Glanz (1988), provides a helpful approach to understanding the many factors that shape treatment access and recovery. This model identifies five interconnected levels of influence: intrapersonal, interpersonal, organizational, community, and policy. Each level represents a different layer of barriers or support that can affect someone's ability to seek, access, and continue treatment for OUD. These levels are not isolated; instead, they overlap and influence one another in ways that often complicate the treatment process. For example, a person's struggle with stigma may involve feelings of shame, negative experiences with healthcare providers, and institutional policies that limit care (Bielenberg et al. 2021; McCurry et al. 2023). It may also extend to broader social and legal challenges such as unstable or unsafe housing, employment discrimination, loss of child custody, involvement with the criminal justice system, or restrictive family law policies (Cohen et al. 2022; CDC 2025b). The sections that follow explore the key barriers affecting individuals with OUD and the systems that shape their treatment experiences through the lens of the ecological model of health behavior (Fig. 9.1).

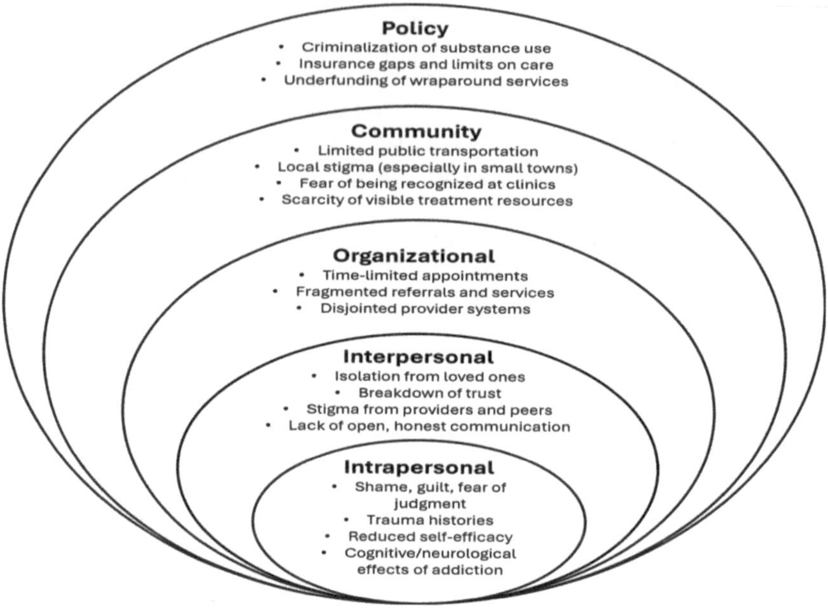

Fig. 9.1 Ecological model illustrating barriers to OUD treatment. Adapted from McLeroy et al.'s (1988) ecological model of health behavior

9.2.1 *Intrapersonal-Level Barriers*

At the intrapersonal level of the ecological model, barriers to treatment for OUD are often rooted in deeply personal struggles such as shame, fear, trauma histories, and the neurological impacts of OUD itself (Luoma et al. 2007; Bielenberg et al. 2021). These internal barriers are invisible to others but can present some of the most significant obstacles to recovery.

Stigma and fear of judgment are among the most pervasive intrapersonal barriers. One mother described her overwhelming fear of disclosing her OUD: "I was worried if I told the doctor about my addiction, I'd lose all my children" (Beckham and Anthony 2022, 12). Studies confirm that fear of judgment from healthcare providers and child welfare systems is a major deterrent to seeking treatment, especially for women (van Boekel et al. 2013; Merrick et al. 2018).

Emotional avoidance also plays a central role. One woman in recovery explained, "When you're using, you're literally taking your feelings and suffocating them" (NBC News Left Field 2018, 8:09). Researchers have found that many individuals with OUD use substances to self-medicate trauma, anxiety, and depression—further entrenching their dependence (Kocherlakota 2014; Garland et al. 2019).

Neurological changes caused by chronic opioid use can further complicate recovery by impairing decision-making and increasing compulsive behaviors (Substance Abuse and Mental Health Services Administration [SAMHSA] 2016; Volkow et al. 2016). An individual struggling with relapse described the exhausting cycle of attempting to cease opioid use: "I've tried many times—to get clean and stay abstinent from it ... I wouldn't wish this addiction on my worst enemy. It's probably the hardest thing I have ever been forced to do" (The White House 2018, "David," 0:47).

The cumulative impact of these barriers often leads to profound losses. One woman reflected on the devastating fallout from her addiction: "I lost everything—my children, my house, my home—everything" (The White House 2018, "Michelle," 0:36). These stories corroborate broader research findings indicating that OUD frequently results in severe social, emotional, and financial consequences—losses that deepen isolation and can create seemingly insurmountable barriers to recovery (SAMHSA 2016; Mackey et al. 2020).

9.2.2 Interpersonal-Level Barriers

At the interpersonal level of the ecological model, family members, friends, peers, and healthcare providers play a pivotal role in shaping treatment outcomes for individuals with OUD (Anvari et al. 2022). These relationships often make the difference between connection and isolation, recovery and relapse (Beckham and Anthony 2022).

Isolation is a frequent and pernicious consequence of OUD. Social connections often deteriorate as individuals attempt to conceal their drug use or avoid the judgment of others. One man from Georgia recounted how he withdrew from his social circle: "I dropped all my friends. I didn't do anything but go to work and pop pills" (The White House 2018, "Justin," 1:12). This type of withdrawal may feel protective, but it severs critical sources of emotional support—leaving people alone with their drug problem (Judd et al. 2023; Nguyen et al. 2024). Studies show that weakened social networks are a significant barrier to recovery, with many individuals reporting worsened mental health and reduced motivation to seek treatment (Barry et al. 2009; Cochran et al. 2024).

In the case of self-isolating individuals, families often remain unaware of a loved one's opioid dependence. Even when it is suspected, secrecy and denial frequently prevent open conversations about treatment needs, which strains relationships, erodes trust, creates conflict, and leaves relatives divided over how to respond (McCann and Lubman 2018; Bagley and Beckham 2020). Ashley from Kansas described the unexpected horror of losing her sister to fentanyl: "We were shocked and devastated. We had no idea she was using drugs. The toxicology showed that she died from an analog of fentanyl. She left behind two boys, age 11 and age 13, and I had to tell my own children who are six and eight that their beloved aunt was gone and that was very hard" (The White House 2018, "Ashley," 0:39). Stories like Ashley's are not uncommon, and many families only recognize the severity of opioid use after it is too late (Mackey et al. 2020).

Stigma also emerges in clinical settings, where healthcare providers may unconsciously or even openly express negative judgments about patients with OUD. One woman recalled overhearing her provider say, "Oh, she's just a junkie from around the corner and she'll either come back on a gurney dead or relapse again, so what's the use of getting her clean" (Beckham and Anthony 2022, 13). Such encounters are not outliers. Studies consistently find that stigma from healthcare providers is a major barrier to treatment, leading many patients to delay care, minimize disclosure, or disengage from treatment altogether (van Boekel et al. 2013; Biancarelli et al. 2019; McCurry et al. 2023; Cheetham et al. 2022).

These interpersonal barriers—shrinking social circles, strained family ties, and stigmatizing healthcare encounters—often leave individuals isolated and unsupported. Chris, reflecting on the widespread damage of opioids in his community, remarked, "Addiction sucks. It destroys families, individuals, and communities" (The White House 2018, "Chris," 0:26). His words capture the broad reach of opioid addiction across personal relationships, social networks, and healthcare systems. Together, these narratives and studies illuminate how interpersonal barriers compound the challenges of recovery, reinforcing cycles of isolation and opioid dependence (Barry et al. 2009; Anvari et al. 2022; Cochran et al. 2024).

9.2.3 *Organizational-Level Barriers*

Organizational barriers emerge within healthcare systems, treatment programs, and other institutions where administrative structures, reimbursement models, and service delivery policies directly shape both patient and provider experiences. While these challenges overlap with those at the broader community and policy levels, they create distinct institutional obstacles—often limiting access, fragmenting care, and undermining recovery efforts.

For patients with OUD, institutional hurdles can be the first barriers encountered when seeking healthcare. One individual described her experience bluntly: "I was rejected by two hospitals and several clinics" (Beckham 2019, 14). Strict intake requirements, limited program capacity, and disjointed services often prevent individuals from initiating care (Mackey et al. 2020).

Clinicians face barriers as well. Many describe being forced to prioritize speed over meaningful patient interaction due to productivity demands. One provider explained, "I wish I had more time to talk to my patients about their situation, but I'm expected to move through appointments quickly" (Beckham and Anthony 2022, 17). In some cases, provider compensation is directly tied to the number of patients seen: "Hospital administrators keep up with how many patients a doctor sees ... the doctor's salary is fully connected with how much money they generate" (Beckham and Anthony 2022, 18). These policies often create limitations, preventing the kind of in-depth counseling and coordination that individuals with OUD require (Krebs et al. 2014).

With providers facing perpetual time constraints, community behavioral health services can help fill in the gaps. Unfortunately, behavioral health services that are critical for long-term recovery are frequently poorly integrated and underfunded (Moran et al. 2019). One clinician explained the gap:

> They need behavioral health and they need someone who can talk to them—just to say, you know, "How are you doing? Do you have food? Is somebody at your house ... selling drugs?" Those are the kinds of things that require behavioral health. And it should be paid for, and it's not. (Beckham and Anthony 2022, 20)

However, even when viable referrals are available, systemic limitations frequently undermine their effectiveness. One provider shared, "We need knowledge of resources so that we can talk about them … it's not like you've got time to go out and be like, 'let me go look this up for you'" (Beckham and Anthony 2022, 21).

Transitions of care expose deeper cracks in organizational systems. Changes in insurance, providers, or care settings frequently disrupt treatment at times of heightened vulnerability. Dr. Tara Benjamin, an OB-GYN, described how these changes affect new mothers with opioid use disorder:

> That's kind of the biggest barrier that we have because that transition time is very important. It's a period where they are very stressed out, they're very fatigued, they have a brand-new baby … they also have a risk of postpartum depression … and all of these things are really high risks for relapse … It's such a shame if they end up relapsing in the postpartum period just because they couldn't transition. (Side Effects Public Media 2017, 6:32)

Organizational barriers like these often leave both patients and providers struggling within systems that are disjointed, overstretched, and unable to meet the complex needs of individuals with OUD (Mackey et al. 2020; Beckham and Anthony 2022).

9.2.4 Community-Level Barriers

Individuals with OUD often encounter additional challenges within their communities that impede their recovery efforts. One of the most common and frustrating obstacles is the difficulty of connecting with treatment options. One patient described her struggle to locate support, saying, "I wanted to get clean so bad, but I couldn't find anyone to help" (Krauth 2016, 1:09). This experience is frequently reported by patients and healthcare providers. In many cases, people who are ready to seek treatment simply cannot find a clear path to services within their community. Several studies have documented this lack of accessible information, evidencing that individuals often face confusing or incomplete information about local resources (Mackey et al. 2020; Beckham and Anthony 2022; McCurry et al. 2023). Even healthcare professionals themselves may be unaware of available treatment options in their area, leaving patients with neither referrals nor guidance critical to recovery.

Transportation issues are also frequently noted by healthcare providers who see patients miss appointments or struggle to maintain consistent care because they lack reliable modes of travel. Providers may address this issue through organizational support systems that facilitate ride arrangements, but the problem itself is rooted in broader community conditions. In many rural and underserved areas, patients must travel long distances to access treatment on their own as public transit systems are limited or nonexistent (Bunting et al. 2018; Lister et al. 2020). The National Institutes of Health (NIH) and the American Hospital Association (AHA) identify transportation as a major social determinant of health that can affect access to medical care and behavioral health treatment (Health Research & Educational Trust 2017; Wolfe et al. 2020). In communities without public transit systems, individuals who are ready to pursue recovery may find themselves completely cut off from services simply because they cannot reach them.

At the same time, community stigma looms as a powerful obstacle, particularly in smaller towns where privacy is limited. In close-knit communities, individuals holding highly visible jobs such as healthcare workers, teachers, or clergy often worry that seeking treatment could harm their personal or professional reputations (Bunting et al. 2018; Biancarelli et al. 2019; Judd et al. 2023). The fear of being seen at a treatment center or pharmacy is a deterrent for people from seeking care, even when they are otherwise motivated to act.

Jackie, a nurse living in a small town, described the immense shame that kept her from accessing local care: "There was no way I was going to one of my local doctors here," she said. "I work in the healthcare business … you kind of know everyone in a small town, so it just wasn't going to happen" (Bright Heart Health 2024, 0:04). For healthcare professionals like Jackie, the fear of being seen and judged compounds the emotional burden of addiction, further isolating them and delaying treatment. Such stories reflect a broader reality faced by many in rural communities, where stigma doesn't just shape perception, it limits access to care.

Compounding these difficulties, some neighborhoods face environmental conditions that intensify the feeling of hopelessness and normalize drug use. In areas where drug overdoses and discarded needles are common sights, constant exposure to these triggers can make addiction feel inescapable. One resident of Worcester, Massachusetts, described the emotional toll of her surroundings:

> It is very disturbing to walk down Main Street in your own city and see people overdosed in alleyways and see needles littered on the ground and have your child ask what they're for … Politicians don't see the effects on the people that live in those areas that aren't drug addicts, and how it drives some people to drugs anyway because they can't escape it. (The White House 2018, "Sarah," 0:27)

Such conditions not only pose public health risks but also reinforce cycles of trauma and despair for those struggling with addiction and for the community as a whole.

Another challenge many communities face is the lack of consistent education regarding opioid risks and treatment options. In areas without strong public health campaigns or prevention efforts, people may not fully grasp the dangers of opioid use or know where to turn for help. One individual from Michigan described how this lack of prevention education shaped his experience: "There were no commercials or anything telling me what they would do to me. If there was, I wouldn't have ever taken a Vicodin. They are the devil" (The White House 2018, "Chris," 0:39). National public health reports confirm that inconsistent education limits prevention and recovery efforts in many areas (Volkow et al. 2019).

These barriers reveal how deeply the community and local environment can influence prevention, treatment, and recovery related to OUD. Challenges such as limited access to education and services, transportation difficulties, stigma, and environmental factors often overlap in ways that make it extremely difficult for individuals with OUD to maintain or even initiate recovery. These realities continue to shape how people experience the opioid crisis in communities across the country.

9.2.5 Policy-Level Barriers

At the outermost level of the ecological model, local, state, and federal policies profoundly influence the landscape of OUD treatment. While some progress has been made through increased funding and public awareness, many policies continue to reinforce stigma, create bureaucratic hurdles, and restrict the requisite resources for long-term recovery (Terry 2019). These policy-level barriers ripple through all other layers of the ecological model, determining institutional practices, patient-provider relationships, community attitudes, and individual decisions to seek care.

One of the most persistent policy challenges relates to the criminalization of substance abuse, especially among pregnant individuals. Although punitive approaches to substance use during pregnancy have softened in some states, laws in many states still emphasize surveillance and punishment over treatment (Voss et al. 2025). Studies show that fear of criminal charges or child welfare involvement often prevents pregnant individuals from seeking prenatal care or disclosing opioid use, even when treatment services are available (CNN 2017). This chilling effect pushes many into hiding and delays critical interventions at the expense of the health of unborn children.

Health insurance policies present another major obstacle to recovery. Despite Medicaid expansion in some states, many individuals with OUD face coverage gaps, high out-of-pocket costs, or restrictive treatment rules (Mackey et al. 2020). Coverage is often inconsistent for essential services like medication-assisted treatment (MAT) and behavioral health counseling. Pregnant individuals may temporarily qualify for care only to lose it shortly after childbirth, a period when relapse risk is especially high (SAMHSA 2021). Additionally, many insurance plans require prior authorization for OUD medications or limit treatment duration, creating obstacles that can derail recovery efforts (Volkow et al. 2019). Research has shown that these administrative hurdles prevent timely access to care and conflict with clinical guidelines that recommend rapid initiation of treatment (Wakeman and Barnett 2018).

Beyond insurance, broader underinvestment in addiction treatment services leaves many treatment programs under-resourced. Funding restrictions limit the availability of wraparound supports such as housing assistance, transportation vouchers, and peer recovery services, which are essential for sustained recovery (Moran et al. 2019). While MAT is widely recognized as the gold standard of care by agencies such as the CDC, NIH, and SAMHSA, many communities still face shortages of qualified providers and programs capable of delivering comprehensive care (SAMHSA 2021).

As journalist Sky Dylan-Dobbins explained in a report on opioid addiction, "medication-assisted treatment has been embraced by every major health agency. So what's the holdup in making it the standard? The answer, far too often, is stigma baked into policies and funding priorities" (NBC News Left Field 2018, 4:09).

Structural issues also affect healthcare providers. Many clinicians report that restrictive policies, limited reimbursement, and the threat of regulatory scrutiny deter them from offering MAT or related services (Barry et al. 2009). These issues not only limit the availability of care but also undermine the quality of communication between providers and patients, making it more difficult to develop trusting, supportive relationships.

Ultimately, these policy-level barriers shape every facet of OUD treatment and recovery. When policies promote punishment over prevention, restrict insurance access, or limit funding to essential services, they contribute to a treatment system that is fragmented, inequitable, and difficult to access and navigate. These challenges illustrate how policy decisions can undermine treatment and recovery efforts, reinforcing the need for more compassionate, evidence-based approaches that align with the realities of addiction and the needs of those seeking care and recovery.

9.3 Applying Patient-Centered Communication and Navigation Across the Ecological Model

Insights from individuals struggling with OUD elucidate many of the obstacles they face on the road to recovery. While many individuals express a strong desire to stop using opioids, they frequently encounter overwhelming barriers such as fear, stigma, and systemic challenges that stand in their way (Bunting et al. 2018; Mackey et al. 2020). As the earlier testimonials show, these barriers often create uncertainty. Many people are left unsure of where to turn, how to pay for care, or whether any program will accept them (Moran et al. 2019; Cheetham et al. 2022). Their stories make it clear that recovery is not simply a matter of willpower. Instead, it requires sustained, coordinated, and compassionate support (Luoma et al. 2007; Volkow et al. 2016).

These accounts demonstrate that for recovery to succeed, it is necessary to address many interwoven barriers at the same time (Bielenberg et al. 2021; Beckham and Anthony 2022). There is no single solution to OUD. Rather, the only viable path forward is through a comprehensive strategy that removes barriers, reduces stigma, and replaces fear with hope (Terry 2019). Communication serves as the critical thread that binds these efforts together (Street 2003). It is the tool that disrupts negative patterns and fosters trust, understanding, and motivation (Epstein and Street 2007). Effective communication at the individual, organizational, and community levels can help dismantle stigma, reduce confusion, and encourage long-term engagement with care (Beckham and Anthony 2022).

Patient-centered communication (PCC) and patient navigation stand out as strategies that help mitigate barriers across ecological levels. PCC specifically addresses the relational and informational needs that arise within clinical encounters, promoting mutual respect and clarity between patient and provider (Epstein and Street 2007). Patient navigators operate outside those encounters, coordinating care, building trust, and offering practical support in patients' daily lives (Freeman 2004). Together, these approaches offer a powerful and comprehensive framework to support people suffering from OUD as they navigate their recovery journeys.

9.4 The Role of Patient-Centered Communication (PCC) in OUD Care

PCC was originally developed to improve cancer care by addressing the emotional, informational, and logistical challenges patients and families often face throughout treatment (Epstein and Street 2007; Mazor et al. 2013). The communication model identifies six essential functions of effective communication: fostering healing relationships, exchanging information effectively, responding to emotions, supporting quality decision-making, managing uncertainty, and enabling self-care (Epstein and Street 2007, 2011).

Although PCC originated in the context of cancer care, it has been widely adapted to the care of other complex health conditions, including OUD. Individuals with OUD frequently encounter fragmented services, stigma, and mistrust within healthcare systems (McGinty et al. 2015; Wakeman and Barnett 2018; Biancarelli et al. 2019). PCC is particularly beneficial for these individuals because it promotes empathy, mutual respect, and collaborative engagement in treatment. By fostering clear communication and shared decision-making, PCC can empower patients to approach their recovery with greater confidence and dignity (Epstein and Street 2007; Barry et al. 2009).

9.4.1 Fostering Healing Relationships

Many individuals with OUD report that healthcare encounters leave them feeling judged or dismissed. For these patients, cultivating a healing relationship is often the first step toward rebuilding trust. Providers who take the time to listen, show empathy, and work collaboratively with patients can help reverse the sense of rejection that many people have experienced (Bielenberg et al. 2021; McCurry et al. 2023). As Dr. Catherine Livingston explained, opioid dependence, like diabetes, should be treated as a chronic disease. She emphasized that patients should not be denied care for struggling with OUD, just as a diabetic patient would never be refused treatment (NBC News Left Field 2018). One woman described how meaningful it was to have a cohesive care team working in unison to support her recovery, stating, “It was really unique having all the doctors come together and work as a team to help one single person” (Athena Health 2016, 1:20).

9.4.2 *Exchanging Information Effectively*

The ability to exchange information clearly and compassionately impacts how patients experience their care. For many people navigating OUD treatment, medical jargon, emotional stress, and cognitive overload make it difficult to absorb complex information (Drossman and Ruddy 2020; McCurry et al. 2023). Effective information exchange happens when providers explain treatment options in plain language, paced according to the patient’s readiness to process the information. Dobrozsi and colleagues (2019) have noted that emotional readiness can strongly influence a patient’s ability to understand medical information. One patient described how her provider made a difference by taking time to explain her treatment options in everyday language, outlining what each plan involved and how it might affect her, which helped her feel more confident and comfortable with her care (The Ohio State University Wexner Medical Center 2017).

9.4.3 *Responding to Emotions*

Addiction takes a heavy emotional toll, and patients often carry intense feelings of shame, guilt, and fear. This is why responding to emotions plays such a critical role in PCC. Rather than ignoring these feelings, providers who validate and acknowledge them help create a safer, more compassionate treatment environment (Luoma et al. 2007; Bunting et al. 2018). Dr. Livingston stressed that addiction fundamentally alters brain chemistry, making intensive, empathetic treatment essential. Her perspective reinforces the need to approach addiction as a serious health condition, rather than as a personal failing (NBC News Left Field 2018). Patients often highlight how impactful it is to have providers who listen without judgment and support them emotionally, especially when they are navigating difficult decisions or setbacks (Beckham and Anthony 2022).

9.4.4 *Supporting Quality Decision-Making*

Making difficult treatment decisions is a part of the OUD recovery process. Patients must weigh complex options regarding medications, withdrawal management, and lifestyle adjustments. Many feel unsure about the risks and benefits of their choices, making it essential for providers to guide them through these decisions in a supportive and respectful manner (Barry et al. 2009; Mackey et al. 2020). Shared decision-making ensures that patients' values and preferences are considered, even as providers offer clear, evidence-based recommendations (Elwyn et al. 2012; Thorne et al. 2014). One patient described how a provider helped her feel empowered during a pivotal moment in her care by explaining the risks of quitting abruptly while also offering immediate medication support (Side Effects Public Media 2017).

9.4.5 *Managing Uncertainty*

Fear of the unknown is common among patients recovering from OUD. Uncertainty about relapses, withdrawal symptoms, and treatment success can create significant anxiety (Barry et al. 2009; Moran et al. 2019). Providers who proactively address these concerns and offer clear, honest communication can help ease these fears. Research shows that unaddressed uncertainty is a frequent cause of emotional distress and communication breakdowns in healthcare settings (Mazor et al. 2013; Street et al. 2019). Discussing potential challenges and offering concrete plans for managing them can help patients feel more prepared and resilient, even when recovery does not follow a predictable path (Wakeman and Barnett 2018).

9.4.6 *Enabling Self-Care*

Treating OUD within the walls of a clinic is only one part of the process. Since many individuals with OUD face social and environmental challenges such as housing instability, unemployment, and limited support networks (Lister et al. 2020; Bielenberg et al. 2021), it is incumbent on providers to equip patients with strategies to manage their health beyond the clinic. A key function of PCC is enabling self-care by preparing patients to deal with stressors and triggers that most often occur at home, at work, and in their communities. Providers support this process by connecting patients to community-based services such as treatment programs, housing or transportation assistance, and peer support groups, while also teaching harm-reduction techniques and offering guidance on managing cravings and stress. Together, these efforts set the stage for long-term recovery (Wakeman and Barnett 2018; Mackey et al. 2020).

9.5 The Role of Patient Navigation in OUD Care

Patient navigation plays a critical role in addressing barriers that remain even after PCC efforts are in place. While PCC provides the foundation for empathetic and collaborative care, time limitations, systemic constraints, and complex patient needs often prevent healthcare providers from helping patients overcome all the challenges the patients face during clinical visits. In these situations, patient navigators serve as trusted allies who extend the core principles of PCC beyond the clinic and into the broader healthcare system.

Patient navigation's root is in cancer care, where it was developed to address the logistical, financial, and systemic hurdles that underserved patients encountered from diagnosis through treatment (Freeman and Rodriguez 2011). Initially formalized under the National Cancer Institute's Patient Navigation Research Program (PNRP), the service was designed to guide vulnerable individuals (e.g., those confronting abnormal cancer screenings) through the complex healthcare system (Freeman 2004; Freund et al. 2008). Over time, patient navigation proved so effective that it expanded well beyond oncology. Studies link patient navigation services to more efficient healthcare delivery and improved patient outcomes across a range of medical conditions (Desimini et al. 2011; Natale-Pereira et al. 2011; Kline et al. 2019).

As the service expanded beyond cancer care, patient navigation started to be carried out by two primary types of navigators, distinguished by their professional training and scope of responsibility. Nurse navigators are registered nurses (RNs) with clinical expertise to educate patients, explain diagnoses and treatment options, coordinate care, and address medical concerns (Oncology Nursing Society 2017). Lay navigators, by contrast, are trained nonprofessionals who focus on reducing nonclinical barriers by arranging transportation, providing appointment reminders, and/or connecting patients to community resources (Freund et al. 2014; Oncology Nursing Society 2017). Patients may have different navigators during their treatment and recovery process depending on their needs and the resources available. Regardless of role, all patient navigators share the same goals: to reduce barriers that threaten to overwhelm patients and to keep them engaged in care.

For individuals struggling with OUD, patient navigation can be particularly transformative (Anvari et al. 2022; McCurry et al. 2023). Much like cancer patients, people with OUD often face fragmented healthcare systems, emotional distress, and logistical barriers including unreliable transportation, insurance lapses, and unstable housing (Carroll et al. 2010; Wakeman and Barnett 2018; Moran et al. 2019). Many providers acknowledge they lack the time, institutional support, or community connections necessary to address these challenges (Beckham and Anthony 2022). One provider noted that up to half of their patients routinely miss appointments because of transportation barriers, demonstrating how easily care can be disrupted by what might seem like minor obstacles.

Patient navigators fill these gaps in provider care by supporting continuity of care and reinforcing the relational and informational aspects of PCC (Freund et al. 2014). Acting as boundary spanners, they help patients move between providers, appointments, and services. One patient described how her nurse navigator ensured consistent care, stating, "she just made sure that I was at every appointment. The nurse was my advocate, and she was my first phone call if something happened" (Patient 14, Beckham and Anthony 2022, 13). In addition to emotional support, navigators often provide tangible assistance. One patient shared how her nurse navigator provided a gas card and a car seat to ensure she could attend appointments, noting that this kind of help not only addressed transportation barriers but also made her feel genuinely supported during her recovery process (Athena Health 2016). Such interventions can prevent missed care and reduce the risk of relapse or treatment dropout (Bunting et al. 2018; Moran et al. 2019).

Beyond logistical support, patient navigators frequently develop deeper, more trusting relationships with patients than providers can during brief medical visits (Anvari et al. 2022; McCurry et al. 2023). Many patients see navigators not as authority figures but as advocates and supporters who listen without judgment. This emotional connection is pivotal for individuals who carry deep stigma and/or have repeated negative healthcare experiences. One person described how community judgment worsened her drug use, creating a vicious cycle of shame and isolation (The Recovery Village 2020). A supportive navigator can break that cycle by offering empathy and reassurance that recovery is possible. By investing time in understanding patients' lived experiences and fears, navigators can also help elicit sensitive information that providers might otherwise miss. In one case, a nurse practitioner learned of a patient's fear of losing custody and lack of partner support—insights that allowed for a more tailored and effective care plan (Beckham and Anthony 2022).

Navigators also play a vital role in tackling the bureaucratic complexities that so often undermine recovery progress (Bunting et al. 2018; Wakeman and Barnett 2018). For example, they help fill out insurance paperwork, apply for treatment funding, and complete other administrative tasks that patients may struggle to manage, particularly those facing housing instability, limited phone access, or other pressing social needs (Moran et al. 2019). Without this support, many patients may fall through the cracks of a system ill-equipped to accommodate their complex situations (McCurry et al. 2023).

In fragmented systems where patients encounter disjointed care and conflicting messages, navigators offer consistency, accountability, and advocacy (Natale-Pereira et al. 2011; Freund et al. 2014). They bridge gaps between patients and providers, hospitals and communities, and policies and practical realities. By fostering trust, addressing concrete barriers, and amplifying patients' voices, navigators become a living extension of PCC, ensuring that comprehensive, compassionate treatment for OUD is not just an ideal but a reality with tangible impact (Cochran et al. 2024).

9.6 Strategies to Extend PCC and Patient Navigation Across the Ecological Model

According to the ecological model, barriers to OUD treatment exist at multiple levels, from individual struggles to systemic and policy obstacles. As discussed throughout this chapter, PCC and patient navigation can be effective strategies for helping patients overcome these barriers to OUD care and treatment. That said, additional steps are needed to ensure addiction care and treatment is transformed. This section highlights how PCC and patient navigation can be better deployed to foster empathy, trust, access, and long-term recovery at each level of the ecological model.

At the individual and interpersonal levels, integrating PCC principles into professional training is essential. This includes training healthcare providers, mental health counselors, social workers, judges, law enforcement officers, housing managers, and others who interact with individuals with OUD. By emphasizing empathic listening, clarity in messaging, and a recognition of the social contexts that patients inhabit, these stakeholders can help reduce stigma and encourage patients to seek timely care (Bielenberg et al. 2021). For example, policymakers could mandate continuing education programs that highlight trauma-informed communication and cultural competence, thereby ensuring that OUD treatment is consistently approached with respect and understanding (SAMHSA 2016).

At the organizational level, healthcare systems and treatment programs should reevaluate workflow designs and reimbursement models to determine how they can better support meaningful communication (Wakeman and Barnett 2018; Moran et al. 2019). Many providers work under time constraints that preclude in-depth conversations about risks, options, and patient concerns. Allowing for longer appointments, reimbursing motivational interviewing or counseling sessions, and hiring patient navigators to shoulder administrative tasks can ease this burden and enable deeper engagement between patient and provider (Moran et al. 2019; Cochran et al. 2024). In this sense, organizational-level reforms are not just structural but communicative as they create the conditions under which PCC can thrive.

At the community level, communication campaigns should highlight recovery, compassion, and resources instead of using fear appeals that perpetuate stereotypes. Local coalitions, public health agencies, and media outlets can collaborate to create messages that normalize seeking help, emphasize recovery success stories, and direct individuals to available services (McGinty et al. 2015; SAMHSA 2016; Bielenberg et al. 2021). Such campaigns can profoundly shape interpersonal conversations about OUD, replacing blame and fear with empathy and support. By drawing on stories of real patients, these efforts can become powerful vehicles for promoting public awareness and early intervention.

Finally, policy changes must reflect the centrality of communication in sustaining recovery. Extending Medicaid coverage or eliminating cumbersome prior authorization requirements not only has a direct impact on treatment continuity but reduces the "noise" that can overwhelm patient-provider communication (Wakeman and Barnett 2018). When patients no longer face constant fear of losing coverage, they can focus more on discussing progress and concerns with their healthcare team. In tandem, legislatures and regulatory bodies can incentivize the expansion of patient navigation programs, ensuring that individuals struggling with OUD have consistent, well-trained allies to help them interpret clinical guidance, access resources, and maintain a sense of hope throughout the recovery process (Moran et al. 2019; Cochran et al. 2024).

By weaving PCC and patient navigation into every aspect of OUD treatment and prevention, from frontline interactions to the highest levels of policy, we can create a culture in which empathy, evidence, and partnership guide our collective responses (McGinty et al. 2015; Beckham and Anthony 2022). The urgency of the opioid epidemic leaves no room for superficial fixes; rather, it demands a sustained and holistic commitment to changing how we talk about, deliver, and organize care. In the end, these communication-centered strategies do more than lower overdose rates or increase treatment retention—they reaffirm the dignity and worth of every individual affected by OUD.

9.7 Conclusion

Jessica Nickel, President and CEO of the Addiction Policy Forum, stated that "only 10% of people get treatment. Can you imagine if only 10% of Alzheimer's or cancer patients received treatment?" (Nickel 2018). This stark reality underscores the urgency for systemic change. The opioid crisis does more than expose gaps in healthcare; it highlights how we, as a society, listen, respond, and care for those struggling with addiction. Individuals with OUD navigate not only the physiological challenges of substance dependence but also stigma, structural neglect, and emotional isolation (Luoma et al. 2007; Dasgupta et al. 2018).

The ecological model reminds us that these challenges operate at every level, from the intrapersonal shame that prevents disclosure of OUD to the policy constraints that limit insurance coverage. PCC and patient navigation (Freeman 2004; Epstein and Street 2007), rooted in empathy and grounded in evidence, offer more than clinical techniques; they represent a fundamental shift toward recognizing the inherent dignity of every patient. By incorporating PCC principles into all sectors of public life and supporting robust navigation networks, we can build systems that heal instead of harming and ensure that no individual faces recovery alone.

If only 10% of the population with OUD receive treatment, then 90% are still waiting—waiting for a system that sees them, serves them, and believes they are worth saving. The insights in this chapter make one thing clear: we do not face a lack of evidence or understanding, rather a lack of action. PCC and patient navigation are not radical innovations; they are practical, proven responses to a preventable crisis. When built into care at every ecological level, these approaches do more than address addiction; they restore human connection in places where it has long been missing. The path forward is not without challenges, but the cost of inaction is lost lives. The time to build a healthcare system rooted in empathy, equity, and coordinated care is now!

References

Anvari, Morgan S., Mary B. Kleinman, Ebonie C. Massey, et al. 2022. "In Their Mind, They Always Felt Less Than": The Role of Peers in Shifting Stigma as a Barrier to Opioid Use Disorder Treatment Retention. *Journal of Substance Abuse Treatment* 138:108721. https://doi.org/10.1016/j.jsat.2022.108721.

Athena Health. 2016. Pregnant and Addicted to Opioids: A Mother Speaks. YouTube Video. https://youtu.be/6NBNKvYSWPo?si=WwZMxPKOf6KEvMBX.

Bagley, Braden, and Jessica Beckham. 2020. Building Messages for the Opioid Crisis Using the Extended Parallel Process Model. *Qualitative Research Reports in Communication* 22 (1): 47–55. https://doi.org/10.1080/17459435.2020.1836017.

Barry, Declan T., Kevin S. Irwin, Emlyn S. Jones, et al. 2009. Integrating Buprenorphine Treatment Into Office-based Practice: A Qualitative Study. *Journal of General Internal Medicine* 24 (2): 218–225. https://doi.org/10.1007/s11606-008-0881-9.

Beckham, Jessica. 2019. *Patient-Provider Communication Involving Opioid Dependent Expecting Mothers: Determining Factors Impacting Communication*, Paper presented at the Alabama Communication Association Conference, University of Montevallo, Montevallo, AL, July 27.

Beckham, Jessica, and Kathryn E. Anthony. 2022. *Factors Influencing Patient-Clinician Communication Involving Maternal Opioid Addiction through the Lens of Patient-Centered Communication*, Paper presented at the National Communication Association 108th Annual Convention. New Orleans, LA, November 17–20.

Biancarelli, Dea L., Katie B. Biello, Ellen Childs, et al. 2019. Strategies Used by People Who Inject Drugs to Avoid Stigma in Healthcare Settings. *Drug and Alcohol Dependence* 198:80–86. https://doi.org/10.1016/j.drugalcdep.2019.01.037.

Bielenberg, Jennifer, Gabrielle Swisher, Anna Lembke, and Nancy A. Haug. 2021. A Systematic Review of Stigma Interventions for Providers who Treat Patients with Substance Use Disorders. *Journal of Substance Abuse Treatment* 131:108486. https://doi.org/10.1016/j.jsat.2021.108486.

Boekel, Van, C. Leonieke, Evelien P. Brouwers, Jaap van Weeghel, and Henk F. Garretsen. 2013. Stigma Among Health Professionals Towards Patients with Substance Use Disorders and its Consequences for Healthcare Delivery: Systematic Review. *Drug and Alcohol Dependence* 131 (1–2): 23–35. https://doi.org/10.1016/j.drugalcdep.2013.02.018.

Bright Heart Health. 2024. Jackie's Story: A Nurse's Journey Through Opioid Addiction and Recovery. YouTube Video, 3:13, February 6. https://www.youtube.com/watch?v=U2X3HDYNKj8.

Bunting, Amanda M., Carrie B. Oser, Michele Staton, Katherine S. Eddens, and Hannah Knudsen. 2018. Clinician Identified Barriers to Treatment for Individuals in Appalachia with Opioid Use Disorder Following Release from Prison: A Social Ecological Approach. *Addiction Science & Clinical Practice* 13 (1): 23. https://doi.org/10.1186/s13722-018-0124-2.

Carroll, Jennifer K., Sharon G. Humiston, Sean C. Meldrum, et al. 2010. Patients' Experiences with Navigation for Cancer Care. *Patient Education and Counseling* 80 (2): 241–247. https://doi.org/10.1016/j.pec.2009.10.024.

Centers for Disease Control and Prevention. 2024. *Understanding the Opioid Overdose Epidemic. Overdose Prevention.* https://www.cdc.gov/overdose-prevention/about/understanding-the-opioid-overdose-epidemic.html.

Centers for Disease Control and Prevention. 2025a. CDC Reports Decline in U.S. Drug Overdose Deaths. *CDC Newsroom.* https://www.cdc.gov/media/releases/2025/2025-cdc-reports-decline-in-us-drug-overdose-deaths.html.

Centers for Disease Control and Prevention. 2025b. *Stigma: Beyond the Numbers. StopOverdose.* https://www.cdc.gov/stop-overdose/stigma-reduction/stigma-beyond-the-numbers.html.

Cheetham, Ali, Louisa Picco, Anthony Barnett, Dan I. Lubman, and Suzanne Nielsen. 2022. The Impact of Stigma on People with Opioid Use Disorder, Opioid Treatment, and Policy. *Substance Abuse and Rehabilitation* 13:1–12. https://doi.org/10.2147/SAR.S304566.

CNN. 2017. Getting Clean While Pregnant. https://www.cnn.com/2017/05/05/health/opioid-detox-during-pregnancy.

Cochran, Gerald, Marcela C. Smid, Elizabeth E. Krans, et al. 2024. Patient Navigation for Pregnant Individuals with Opioid Use Disorder: Results of a Randomized Multi-Site Pilot Trial. *Addiction* 119 (3): 544–556. https://doi.org/10.1111/add.16364.

Cohen, Aliza, Sheila P. Vakharia, Julie Netherland, and Kassandra Frederique. 2022. How the War on Drugs Impacts Social Determinants of Health Beyond the Criminal Legal System. *Annals of Medicine* 54 (1): 2024–2038. https://doi.org/10.1080/07853890.2022.2100926.

Dasgupta, Nabarun, Leo Beletsky, and Daniel Ciccarone. 2018. Opioid Crisis: No Easy Fix to Its Social and Economic Determinants. *American Journal of Public Health* 108 (2): 182–186. https://doi.org/10.2105/AJPH.2017.304187.

Desimini, Esther Muscari, Janine A. Kennedy, Meg F. Helsley, Karen Shiner, Chris Denton, Toni T. Rice, Barbara Stannard, Patrick W. Farrell, Peter A. Marmerstein, and Margaret G. Lewis. 2011. "Making the Case for Nurse Navigators: Benefits, Outcomes, and Return on Investment." *Oncology Issues* 26(5): 26–33. https://doi.org/10.1080/10463356.2011.11883604.

Drossman, Douglas A., and Johannah Ruddy. 2020. Improving Patient-Provider Relationships to Improve Health Care. *Clinical Gastroenterology and Hepatology* 18 (7): 1417–1426. https://doi.org/10.1016/j.cgh.2019.12.007.

Elwyn, Glyn, Dominick Frosch, Richard Thomson, et al. 2012. Shared Decision Making: A Model for Clinical Practice. *Journal of General Internal Medicine* 27 (10): 1361–1367. https://doi.org/10.1007/s11606-012-2077-6.

Epstein, Ronald M., and Richard L. Street Jr. 2007. *Patient-Centered Communication in Cancer Care: Promoting Healing and Reducing Suffering*. National Cancer Institute, NIH Publication No. 07-6225. Bethesda, MD.

Epstein, Ronald M., and Richard L. Street Jr. 2011. The Values and Value of Patient-Centered Care. *The Annals of Family Medicine* 9 (2): 100–103. https://doi.org/10.1370/afm.1239.

Freeman, Harold P. 2004. A Model Patient Navigation Program: Breaking down Barriers to Ensure That All Individuals with Cancer Receive Timely Diagnosis and Treatment. *Oncology Issues* 19 (5): 44–46. https://doi.org/10.1080/10463356.2004.11884227.

Freeman, Harold P., and Rian L. Rodriguez. 2011. History and principles of patient navigation. *Cancer* 117 (S15): 3539–3542. https://doi.org/10.1002/cncr.26262.

Freund, Karen M., Tracy A. Battaglia, Elizabeth Calhoun, Donald J. Dudley, Kevin Fiscella, Electra Paskett, Peter C. Raich, Richard G. Roetzheim, and Patient Navigation Research Program Group. 2008. National Cancer Institute Patient Navigation Research Program: methods, protocol, and measures. *Cancer* 113(12): 3391–3399. https://doi.org/10.1002/cncr.23960.

Freund, Karen M., Tracy A. Battaglia, Elizabeth Calhoun, et al. 2014. Impact of Patient Navigation on Timely Cancer Care: The Patient Navigation Research Program. *Journal of the National Cancer Institute* 106 (6): https://doi.org/10.1093/jnci/dju115.

Garland, Eric L., Matthew O. Howard, Brett Froeliger, Patrick Finan, and Michael R. Riquino. 2019. Neurophysiological and Behavioral Mechanisms of Mindfulness-Oriented Recovery Enhancement for Chronic Pain and Opioid

Misuse. *Current Pain and Headache Reports* 23 (8): 1–9. https://doi.org/10.1007/s11916-019-0804-6.

Health Research & Educational Trust. 2017. *Social Determinants of Health Series: Transportation and the Role of Hospitals*. Chicago: Health Research & Educational Trust. https://www.aha.org/transportation.

Judd, Hailey, Cristian L. Meier, Ashley C. Yaugher, Emma Campbell, and Kandice Atismé-Bevins. 2023. Opioid Use Disorder Stigma Reduction Through Story Telling Narrative and Sharing: A Qualitative Review and Lessons Learned. *International Journal of Mental Health and Addiction* 21 (1): 468–483. https://doi.org/10.1007/s11469-021-00606-y.

Kline, Ronald M., Gabrielle B. Rocque, Elizabeth A. Rohan, Kris A. Blackley, Cynthia A. Cantril, Mandi L. Pratt-Chapman, Howard A. Burris, and Lawrence N. Shulman. 2019. Patient Navigation in Cancer: The Business Case to Support Clinical Needs. *Journal of Oncology Practice* 15(11): 585–590. https://doi.org/10.1200/JOP.19.00230.

Kocherlakota, Pradeep. 2014. Neonatal Abstinence Syndrome. *Pediatrics* 134 (2): e547–e561. https://doi.org/10.1542/peds.2013-3524.

Krauth, Dan. 2016. Pregnant & Addicted. YouTube Video. NBC 6 South Florida. https://youtu.be/GXJnMt9fazs.

Krebs, Erin E., Alicia A. Bergman, Jessica M. Coffing, Steffanie R. Campbell, Richard M. Frankel, and Marianne S. Matthias. 2014. Barriers to Guideline-Concordant Opioid Management in Primary Care—A qualitative study. *The Journal of Pain* 15 (11): 1148–1155. https://doi.org/10.1016/j.jpain.2014.08.006.

Lister, Jamey J., Addie Weaver, Jennifer D. Ellis, Joseph A. Himle, and David M. Ledgerwood. 2020. A Systematic Review of Rural-Specific Barriers to Medication Treatment for Opioid Use Disorder in the United States. *The American Journal of Drug and Alcohol Abuse* 46 (3): 273–288. https://doi.org/10.1080/00952990.2019.1694536.

Luoma, Jason B., Michael P. Twohig, Thomas Waltz, et al. 2007. An Investigation of Stigma in Individuals Receiving Treatment for Substance Abuse. *Addictive Behaviors* 32 (7): 1331–1346. https://doi.org/10.1016/j.addbeh.2006.09.008.

Lynn, Rachael R., and J. L. Galinkin. 2018. Naloxone Dosage for Opioid Reversal: Current Evidence and Clinical Implications. *Therapeutic Advances in Drug Safety* 9 (1): 63–88. https://doi.org/10.1177/2042098617744161.

Mackey, Katherine, Stephanie Veazie, Johanna Anderson, Donald Bourne, and Kim Peterson. 2020. Barriers and Facilitators to the Use of Medications for Opioid Use Disorder: A Rapid Review. *Journal of General Internal Medicine* 35 (S3): 954–963. https://doi.org/10.1007/s11606-020-06257-4.

Mazor, Kathleen M., Winifred L. Malone, John D. Gallagher, and Robert S. Roblin. 2013. Communicating Effectively About Uncertainty in Cancer

Care. *Patient Education and Counseling* 90 (3): 354–360. https://doi.org/10.1016/j.pec.2012.06.003.

McCann, Terence V., and Dan I. Lubman. 2018. Help-Seeking Barriers and Facilitators for Affected Family Members of a Relative with Alcohol and Other Drug Misuse: A Qualitative Study. *Journal of Substance Abuse Treatment* 93:7–14. https://doi.org/10.1016/j.jsat.2018.07.005.

McCurry, Mary K., Shannon Avery-Desmarais, Monika Schuler, Mirinda Tyo, Jennifer Viveiros, and Brianna Kauranen. 2023. Perceived Stigma, Barriers, and Facilitators Experienced by Members of the Opioid Use Disorder Community When Seeking Healthcare. *Journal of Nursing Scholarship* 55 (3): 701–710. https://doi.org/10.1111/jnu.12837.

McGinty, Emma E., Howard H. Goldman, Bernice Pescosolido, and Colleen L. Barry. 2015. Portraying Mental Illness and Drug Addiction as Treatable Health Conditions: Effects of a Randomized Experiment on Stigma and Discrimination. *Social Science & Medicine* 126:73–85. https://doi.org/10.1016/j.socscimed.2014.12.010.

McLeroy, Kenneth R., Daniel Bibeau, Allan Steckler, and Karen Glanz. 1988. An Ecological Perspective on Health Promotion Programs. *Health Education Quarterly* 15 (4): 351–377. https://doi.org/10.1177/109019818801500401.

Merrick, Melissa T., Derek C. Ford, Katie A. Ports, and Angie S. Guinn. 2018. Prevalence of Adverse Childhood Experiences from the 2011–2014 Behavioral Risk Factor Surveillance System in 23 States. *JAMA Pediatrics* 172 (11): 1038–1044. https://doi.org/10.1001/jamapediatrics.2018.2537.

Moran, Garrett, Hannah Knudsen, and Caroline Snyder. 2019. Psychosocial Supports in Medication-Assisted Treatment: Recent Evidence and Current Practice. In *Psychosocial Supports in Medication-Assisted Treatment: Site Visit Findings and Conclusions, Appendix B*. Washington, DC: Department of Health and Human Services. https://aspe.hhs.gov/basic-report/psychosocial-supports-medication-assisted-treatment-site-visit-findings-and-conclusions.

Natale-Pereira, Ana, Kimberly R. Enard, Lucinda Nevarez, and Lovell A. Jones. 2011. The Role of Patient Navigators in Eliminating Health Disparities. *Cancer* 117 (S15): 3541–3550. https://doi.org/10.1002/cncr.26264.

National Academy for State Health Policy. 2023. Understanding Opioid Settlement Spending Plans Across States: Key Components and Approaches. *Last modified January*17:2023.https://nashp.org/understanding-opioid-settlement-spending-plans-across-states-key-components-and-approaches/.

NBC News Left Field. 2018. Reversing the Stigma of Opioid Addiction. YouTube Video. https://youtu.be/GeOmKACjnpY.

Nguyen, Cecilia M., Grace Kubiak, Neil Dixit, Staci A. Young, and John R. Hayes. 2024. Evaluating Barriers to Opioid Use Disorder Treatment from Patients' Perspectives. *PRiMER: Peer-Reviewed Reports in Medical Education Research* 8:11. https://doi.org/10.22454/PRiMER.2024.458349.

Nickel, Jessica. 2018. Opioid Epidemic, Day Two. In *C-SPAN Video Library*. C-SPAN. https://www.c-span.org/program/house-committee/opioid-epidemic-day-two/499771?442923/opioid-crisis-day-hearing#!

Oncology Nursing Society. 2017. Oncology Nurse Navigator Core Competencies. Pittsburgh, PA. https://www.ons.org/oncology-nurse-navigator-competencies.

Payne, Emily R., Sharon Stancliff, Kirsten Rowe, Jason A. Christie, and Michael W. Dailey. 2024. Comparison of Administration of 8-Milligram and 4-Milligram Intranasal Naloxone by Law Enforcement During Response to Suspected Opioid Overdose—New York, March 2022–August 2023. *Morbidity and Mortality Weekly Report* 73 (5): 110–113. https://doi.org/10.15585/mmwr.mm7305a4.

Side Effects Public Media. 2017. Fighting an Addiction While Pregnant. YouTube Video. https://www.youtube.com/watch?v=UrXUfB94vhc.

Street Jr., Richard L. 2003. Communication in Medical Encounters: An Ecological Perspective. In *The Routledge Handbook of Health Communication*, edited by Teresa L. Thompson, Alicia M. Dorsey, Katherine I. Miller, and Roxanne Parrott. Mahwah, NJ: Lawrence Erlbaum Associates.

Street, Richard L., Erica Spears, Sarah Madrid, and Kathleen M. Mazor. 2019. Cancer survivors' experiences with breakdowns in patient-centered communication. *Psycho-Oncology* 28(2): 423–429. https://doi.org/10.1002/pon.v28.210.1002/pon.4963.

Substance Abuse and Mental Health Services Administration. 2021. Medications for Opioid Use Disorder: For Healthcare and Addiction Professionals, Policymakers, Patients, and Families. In *Treatment Improvement Protocol (TIP) Series 63, Full Document*. U.S. Department of Health and Human Services. https://library.samhsa.gov/sites/default/files/pep21-02-01-002.pdf.

Substance Abuse and Mental Health Services Administration, and Office of the Surgeon General. 2016. Chapter 7 Vision for the Future: A Public Health Approach. In *Facing Addiction in America: The Surgeon General's Report on Alcohol, Drugs, and Health*. Washington, DC: Department of Health and Human Services. https://www.ncbi.nlm.nih.gov/books/NBK424861/.

Terry, Nicolas. 2019. From Health Policy to Stigma and Back Again: The Feedback Loop Perpetuating the Opioid Crisis. *Utah Law Review* 2019 (4): 785–809.

The Ohio State University Wexner Medical Center. 2017. How Ohio State's STEPP Clinic Helps Pregnant Women with Addiction. YouTube Video. https://youtu.be/JufVu73qxtY.

The Recovery Village. 2020. Recovering Mother Talks About Opioid Use During Pregnancy, Facebook Watch video. https://www.facebook.com/watch/?v=777926786048692.

The White House. 2018. *Opioids: The Crisis Next Door*. https://crisisnextdoor.gov.

Thorne, Sally T., Gregory Hislop, Charmaine Kim-Sing, Valerie Oglov, John L. Oliffe, and Kelli I. Stajduhar. 2014. Changing communication needs and preferences across the cancer care trajectory: insights from the patient perspective. *Supportive Care in Cancer* 22(4): 1009–1015. https://doi.org/10.1007/s00520-013-2056-4.

Volkow, Nora D., George F. Koob, and Thomas McLellan. 2016. Neurobiologic Advances from the Brain Disease Model of Addiction. *New England Journal of Medicine* 374 (4): 363–371. https://doi.org/10.1056/NEJMra1511480.

Volkow, Nora D., Emily B. Jones, Emily B. Einstein, and Eric M. Wargo. 2019. Prevention and Treatment of Opioid Misuse and Addiction: A Review. *JAMA Psychiatry* 76 (2): 208–216. https://doi.org/10.1001/jamapsychiatry.2018.3126.

Voss, Maren W., Marcela C. Smid, Julie C. Herrick, et al. 2025. A Scoping Review of Community Harm Reduction Strategies for Maternal and Fetal Opioid Impacts: Implications for Policy. *Substance Use & Addiction Journal* 46:3. https://doi.org/10.1177/29767342241312486.

Wakeman, Sarah E., and Michael L. Barnett. 2018. Primary Care and the Opioid-Overdose Crisis-Buprenorphine Myths and Realities. *New England Journal of Medicine* 379 (1): 1–4. https://doi.org/10.1056/NEJMp1802741.

Wolfe, Mary K., Noreen C. McDonald, and G. Mark Holmes. 2020. Transportation Barriers to Health Care in the United States: Findings From the National Health Interview Survey 1997–2017 *American Journal of Public Health* 110(6): 815–822. https://doi.org/10.2105/AJPH.2020.305579.

CHAPTER 10

The (Mis)alignment of Narcotics Anonymous and the Communication Theory of Resilience

Brooke H. Wolfe and Elizabeth A. Hintz

10.1 Introduction

Meeting the aims of this edited collection on the role of communication in combatting the opioid crisis, our chapter focuses on communication concerning opioid use disorder (OUD). Specifically, this chapter answers the following question, "How do the recommendations of the mutual support organization Narcotics Anonymous (NA) align (or misalign) with the communicative resilience processes proposed by communication theory of resilience (CTR)?" A cornerstone of NA is its 12-step program, comprised of a series of phases people battling OUD and seeking recovery must follow in a group support setting (Narcotics Anonymous World Services [NAWS] 2025). Mutual support organizations, including NA, are central to addiction recovery in the United States even though their

B. H. Wolfe (✉)
Department of Communication, Michigan State University, East Lansing, MI, USA
e-mail: wolfebro@msu.edu

E. A. Hintz
Department of Communication, University of Connecticut, Storrs, CT, USA
e-mail: Elizabeth.hintz@uconn.edu

X. Cao (ed.), *Fighting the Opioid Crisis with Communication*,
https://doi.org/10.1007/978-3-032-31162-7_10

programs have been criticized for their rigid (yet nondenominational) religious dogmatism, lack of professional facilitation, one-size-fits-all approach to addiction and recovery, use of stigmatizing terms (e.g., "addict"), and unknown efficacy rates.

This chapter examines how the 12-step program outlined by NA both maps onto and neglects to integrate the six resilience processes outlined by the CTR for people with OUD (Buzzanell 2010, 1–14). We will apply the CTR to examine how NA implores people with OUD to (not) enact the six specific communicative processes theorized to facilitate sense-making and rebuild following a disruptive trigger event—that is, OUD in this case (Buzzanell 2019, 65–88). We argue that the CTR is well-suited for examining the resilience-promoting communicative processes proposed by NA, as both the CTR and NA implicitly affirm that all people can build resilience. Resilience is defined by the CTR as the process of reintegrating into life after a difficult experience. This broad definition of resilience assumes that anyone can enact resilience rather than positioning resilience as an inherent trait or attribute that is available to only some people. This assumption makes resilience accessible to a larger audience given that anyone is argued to be able to build communicative resilience through interpersonal connection and mutual support in a group setting.

The resilience-promoting communication processes outlined by the CTR include: (a) *crafting normalcy*, creating, maintaining, or adapting existing routines that work to make things feel normal again; (b) *foregrounding productive action while backgrounding negative feelings*, where an individual emphasizes beneficial activities like hobbies instead of focusing on negative emotions; (c) *affirming identity anchors*, when an individual uses communication that centers their place in social groups, including their family, community, or college; (d) *maintaining and using communication networks*, when people engage with existing networks or seek to form new connections to attain social resources; and (e) *putting alternative logics to work*, when people find new ways to look at the disruption through humor, reframing, or creative workarounds for the problem. Recently, augmenting these original five processes, researchers have proposed a sixth process—(f) *critiquing and resisting the status quo*, where an individual discusses concerns and problems to push back against the way things are (or have been) that have culminated in or made possible the difficult life event or trigger (Hintz et al. 2021, 371–380).

The 12-step program promoted by NA offers people with OUD a series of principles to follow that are individually enacted and then discussed interpersonally in mutual peer-support meetings. We examine the NA 12-step program and CTR processes within the context of OUD by comparing NA recommendations to the six CTR processes to assess the extent to which the 12-step NA program maps onto the resilience-promoting communication processes outlined by the CTR. Our analysis reveals that some of these CTR processes are directly encouraged by NA (e.g., maintaining and using communication networks, affirming identity anchors), whereas others are implied (e.g., foregrounding productive action, using alternative logics), or currently unaddressed (e.g., critiquing and resisting the status quo). Based on the analysis, we recommend improving the 12-step program to better serve people with OUD through increasing its focus on some CTR processes (e.g., critiquing and resisting the status quo) and decreasing its focus on other processes (e.g., affirming identity anchors such as Christian identity), given the sociocultural complexities of OUD.

In what follows, we first offer an overview of the CTR, including introducing the six resilience-promoting processes identified by the CTR and conceptualizing OUD as a disruptive trigger event. Then, we overview NA, explain its 12-step program, and outline criticisms of the program. Finally, we map the CTR onto the 12-step NA program to identify areas of overlap and divergence before concluding with recommendations for fully integrating some of the CTR resilience-promoting processes into the NA program to improve its effectiveness.

10.2 The Communication Theory of Resilience (CTR)

Resilience is a concept studied by disciplines across the social sciences, yet remains elusive given substantial differences in how it is conceptualized and measured (Afifi 2018, 5–9). Researchers frequently examine resilience as a psychological trait or other inherent capacity that certain people have (e.g., grit, hardiness, perseverance) (Buzzanell and Turner 2003, 27–57). Regardless of the specific conceptualization, a central question across the resilience literature concerns why some people adapt, and even thrive, when confronted with adversity and stressors, whereas others do not. Resilience research has examined factors associated with trait resilience, such as personality, individual experiences, available resources, and social relationship variables, including attachment style. Much of this research suggests that social relationships have a substantial influence on whether someone can bounce back after adversity due, in part, to the provision of (sometimes mutual) social support (Afifi 2018, 27–57; Scharp et al. 2024, 335–361).

Marking a significant divergence from previous trait-based approaches to examining resilience, Buzzanell proposed that resilience can be cultivated by enacting a series of communication processes (Buzzanell 2010, 1–14; Buzzanell 2019, 65–88). Such processes can be either triggered by (reactive resilience) or enacted in response to anticipating and encountering (anticipatory resilience) a complex set of events or circumstances (conceptualized as "trigger events"). Rather than conceptualizing trigger events merely as stressors or adversities, Buzzanell proposed that people experience trigger events (or disruptive life events) that create stress and discomfort as they attempt to create a new normal (Buzzanell 2010). People might enact one or more communication resilience processes in response to those trigger events over time (Buzzanell 2010, 1–14; Buzzanell 2019, 65–88). These trigger events can be acute (e.g., having a one-time medical emergency) or long-lasting (e.g., living with a chronic illness). We herein conceptualize OUD as a disruptive trigger that spurs the enactment of resilience processes. In sum, the CTR includes three central tenets of (a) trigger events, (b) anticipatory and reactive resilience, and (c) communicative processes that aid individuals in controlling, resisting, or navigating life following a disruption (Buzzanell 2019, 65–88).

According to the CTR, resilience is a foundationally communicative process in which people utilize their social networks, interpersonal relationships, and resources (i.e., discursive, economic, material, symbolic) in response to (or in anticipation of) a trigger(s) or disruption(s) (Buzzanell 2010, 1–14; Buzzanell 2018). In other words, the CTR asserts that resilience is fundamentally created through the communication of messages, narratives, and discourse with others. Scholars begin to examine the CTR communication resilience processes by identifying disruptions that people respond to and attempt to rebound from. They then investigate what CTR process(es) are enacted by people experiencing the disruptions (Buzzanell 2019, 65–88). In the remainder of this section, we will explain disruptions (aka trigger events) that activate the CTR communication resilience process(es), elaborate on the six CTR processes, and argue that OUD is a trigger event that activates the enactment of the CTR processes.

10.2.1 Trigger Events

The CTR contends that resilience is enacted through a series of resilience processes in response to trigger event(s) (Buzzanell 2019). In other words, the resilience processes are "activated" by one or more triggering, disruptive life events. A trigger event is a disruption, or set of disturbances, for an individual, group, or community (Buzzanell 2010, 2018, 2019). It "sets human sense-making in motion" and can either happen to (e.g., death, trauma, illness, disaster) or become activated by (e.g., a divorce) individuals and communities (e.g., immigration legislation; Buzzanell 2010, 1–14). Types of trigger events identified in previous work include medical issues and deaths (e.g., addiction), economic issues (e.g., loss of a job), legal issues (e.g., incarceration), and relationship issues (e.g., divorce; Wilson et al. 2021, 478–513). In response to these trigger events, individuals can communicatively construct a new normal using CTR processes (Buzzanell 2019, 65–88). Recent studies have explored the trigger events experienced by specific social groups that activate resilience processes. For instance, Geary et al. (2023) explored the trigger events that HIV-positive men who have sex with men (MSM) report experiencing (Geary et al. 2023, 91–108). The disruptions revealed by their analysis included (a) discrimination for having multiple marginalized identities, (b) isolation, (c) feelings of uncertainty, and (d) shame. In another CTR study, researchers found that migrants to the United States disclosed (a) government obstacles, (b) cultural differences, and (c) physical distance from their families as trigger events that prompted their resilience processes (Scharp et al. 2021, 395–417). These two examples demonstrate how resilience processes can be activated by trigger events unique to certain social groups.

Moreover, trigger events can be related to mundane or once-in-a-lifetime disruptions (Buzzanell 2019, 65–88). Expanding on this notion, Siegenthaler and her colleagues identified four different patterns (that is, linear, cyclical, compounding, and branching) by which trigger events unfold over time (Siegenthaler et al. 2024, 396–417). *Linear* trigger events refer to those occurring in a predictable temporal order and sequence. For example, a chronically ill person experiences and addresses a health challenge, only to have other health challenges arise subsequently. *Cyclical* trigger events are those that are frequent, recurring, and sometimes unpredictable on a day-to-day basis. An example would be day-to-day symptom flares managed by chronically ill people. *Compounding* trigger events occur when multiple, smaller trigger events coalesce into one larger trigger. For example, a chronically ill person becomes homeless due to day-to-day symptom flares and job loss. Finally, *branching* trigger events occur when one (often smaller) trigger leads to multiple new trigger events. For example, starting a new medication leads to severe side effects that result in hospitalization, loss of income, and a strained romantic relationship.

In addition to the patterns in which trigger events unfold and/or are related to one another, researchers have identified other ways of categorizing these events (Scharp et al. 2021, 395–417; Scharp et al. 2022, 1–30; Siegenthaler et al. 2024). For example, Scharp and colleagues conceptualized trigger events as multilayered, meaning that the trigger events are complex in their occurrence and, in some cases, overlap and co-occur to create a suite of trigger events (Scharp et al. 2022, 1–30). Their framework differentiates three types of trigger events—situational, systematic, and overlapping (that is, both situational and systematic). *Situational* trigger events are defined as catalysts that happen to an individual that are not usually pre-existing factors (i.e., reduced contact with friends and family during treatment). In comparison, *systemic* trigger events occur at a societal level and are related to external conditions; moreover, these trigger events are typically pre-existing and enduring (i.e., being unable to afford a recovery program because insurance does not cover the complete cost, making sobriety a financial constraint). Finally, *overlapping* trigger events materialize when individuals have both situational and systemic trigger events intersecting as both personal and societal disruptions (i.e., a person with OUD not being admitted to a hospital because the healthcare system discriminates against patients with various marginalized identities, including, but not limited to, OUD). Systemic and overlapping trigger events can help highlight the hidden costs and obstacles that some encounter when enacting resilience, which could vary across members of communities that have been historically underrepresented and underserved (Harrison 2013, 97–113).

10.2.2 Processes for Enacting Resilience

As detailed, a trigger is an occurrence that activates the enactment of resilience processes. Buzzanell (2010) outlines the original processes that constitute and promote resilience, including: (a) crafting normalcy, (b) foregrounding productive action while backgrounding negative feelings, (c) affirming identity anchors, (d) maintaining and using communication networks, and (e) putting alternative logics to work. Hintz and her colleagues have since added (f) critiquing and resisting the status quo to this list, bringing the total number of CTR processes to six (Hintz et al. 2021).

Crafting normalcy refers to creating, maintaining, or adapting routines to build normalcy following a disruption. An individual can craft normalcy through actively creating new routines or working to return to regular routines. Normality can be constructed via returning to past rituals or learning from the disruption and integrating change into one's schedule. In Buzzanell and Turner's study examining the enactment of family resilience following parental job loss, families kept Friday night dinners, although the restaurant they chose to patronize was less expensive, as well as Saturday morning outings, which were switched to no-cost activities (Buzzanell and Turner 2003). Despite these changes, these practices constructed a new normal for the families following the job loss. These families built resilience by returning to (and adapting) their regular routines. Both activities were ways that family members "explicitly produced a system of meanings that enabled them to maintain the mundane, the regularities in life," which helped the families navigate the economic disruption in addition to returning to ritualized routines (Buzzanell 2010, 3).

Foregrounding productive action while backgrounding negative feelings is a second process in which an individual emphasizes beneficial activities and discursively "plays down" the negativity they might be feeling. This process often involves conscious decision-making and supporting others (Buzzanell 2019, 1–14). The effort to set aside negative emotions in order to create appropriate feelings in any situation can be considerable, especially during traumatic or disastrous times. When enacting this process, people process their emotions following the disruption and reframe the situation linguistically and metaphorically toward one of constrained hopefulness. In Scharp et al.'s (2021) study on first-generation college students who transitioned to online learning during the COVID-19, participants utilized this process by acknowledging that their situation was unlike any educational experience they had encountered before. To respond to this uncertainty, the students crafted new ways to take action by focusing on exceeding academically and getting good grades instead of focusing on the uncertainty of the ongoing public health crisis.

A third process, *affirming identity anchors*, emerges when an individual uses communication that centers their place in the familial, collegial, or community groups in response to a trigger event (Buzzanell 2010, 1–14). Identity anchors are "relatively enduring cluster[s] of identity discourses upon which individuals rely when describing who they are for themselves and in relation to others," and can include religiosity and religious identification (e.g., being a "good Christian"), although this is an aspect less often discussed in current CTR scholarship (Buzzanell 2010, 4).

By affirming identity anchors in tandem with others, people enact what is most meaningful to them in times of difficulty. People may use "discursive resources" that support a particular identity and a set of values that the trigger event may threaten. Hintz and her colleagues (2021) found that healthcare workers centered on an identity-affirming discourse of "all being on the same team" and jointly criticized the lack of personal protective equipment in the early stages of the pandemic. This identity focus appeared in some ways as a counter to healthcare workers' characterization by others as "heroes." They reportedly felt more like "hostages" instead.

Maintaining and using communication networks is a process by which people engage with existing networks, trim unhelpful network connections, or form new networks to attain social resources to assist in navigating a trigger event (Buzzanell 2019, 65–88). This process centers on building and utilizing social capital as essential to enacting resilience. Existing networks allow people to attain resources from connections with others. Alternatively, people also form new networks that can help navigate a trigger event. While discussing the role that a person's social networks may play in resilience processes, Buzzanell (2010) noted that network connections function as "social capital" for those undergoing disruption. Scharp and colleagues likewise described how migrants documented ways in which they used technology to keep in touch with their families still in their home countries while also making new friends in their new city, which helped migrants "garner support and connection" (Scharp et al. 2021, 395–417).

The fifth process, *putting alternative logics to work*, occurs when people find new ways to look at the trigger event via humor or reformulating the experience. Scharp et al. (2021) found that, in the context of migration, constructing alternative logics was particularly "ubiquitous" in their respondents' narratives of moving to the United States. In this case, putting alternative logics to work took two forms: some migrants spoke positively about their migration, whereas others compared their situation to other migrants and focused on the relative ease of their experience. Another example of putting alternative logics to work was identified by Geary et al. (2023), who found that MSM deployed alternative logics by comparing themselves to others who were not faring as well with

HIV. Additionally, the narratives of MSM included reframing their situation (i.e., their HIV diagnosis) as potentially giving them a better life than they would have had otherwise without getting the disease because they learned that they were worthy of love, respect, and acceptance in their personal life and in medical interactions, which were sentiments many did not believe before their diagnosis.

Finally, *critiquing and resisting the status quo* is a process in which people explicitly discuss concerns and problems to push back against the way things are or have been that culminate in the trigger event (Hintz et al. 2021, 371–380). For example, in a study examining how people experience discrimination related to their race, religion, ethnicity, or nationality in their interactions with others, participants critiqued and resisted the status quo by calling out the systemic injustices that supported the conditions that led to their trigger events (Wolfe et al. 2024, 418–456). The systemic injustices targeted by the critiques included racism, antisemitism, xenophobia, and other bias-related inequities. Participants also criticized how institutions, such as media organizations, perpetuated inequalities that negatively impacted their life. More specifically, they pointed out the negative and untrue stereotypes cultivated by popular U.S. media sources that contributed to the inequalities they faced.

Notably, the CTR asserts that resilience is not just about bouncing back (e.g., coping), but about thriving and actively (re)creating a new sense of normal. For this reason, more recent studies have engaged the adaptation-transformation dialectic of the CTR and found that the communication resilience processes outlined by the CTR can be enacted toward both "continuity" and "change" ends (Wilson et al. 2021, 478–513). For instance, the process of "crafting normalcy" could involve both maintaining existing routines (e.g., Sunday family dinner; continuity) and creating new routines (e.g., attending free family events; change) to cultivate a sense that things are normal following a disruption. Maintaining and using communication networks could involve both engaging existing network connections (e.g., asking employed friends to edit a résumé following a job loss; continuity) and creating new network connections (e.g., seeking new contacts in one's field of employment; change). Hence, the communication resilience processes outlined by the CTR can be enacted toward both continuity and change ends depending on the context.

10.2.3 *Opioid Use Disorder (OUD) as a Disruptive Trigger*

According to the CTR (Buzzanell 2010, 2018, 2019), OUD is a disruptive trigger that might spur the enactment of resilience processes. OUD is a treatable chronic disorder, fitting under the previously identified "medical issues and deaths" category of disruptive trigger event types (Wilson et al. 2021, 478–513). Beyond its manifest content as a medical condition, the disorder is also likely a branching trigger as it unfolds over time (Siegenthaler et al. 2024). For instance, the OUD itself could create multiple other trigger events across time, including physical health problems, relationship strain and dissolution, the loss of a job or home, and/or incarceration or drug-related criminal charges. Given that OUD fits the CTR conceptualization of a disruptive trigger, people suffering from OUD would likely benefit from enacting the resilience processes identified by the CTR.

10.3 Narcotics Anonymous (NA) and Its 12-Step Program

Narcotics Anonymous (NA) is a nondenominational nonprofit founded as a recovery program specifically for people using drugs in California in the 1950s. Despite being a U.S.-based organization, as of the writing of this chapter, NA operates in over 144 countries and hosts more than 70,000 weekly meetings (NAWS 2021). Although NA is nondenominational, its 12-step program still calls upon religious ideas (e.g., of "God") and uses religious language in its materials. Inspired by the 12-step program from Alcoholics Anonymous (AA), the NA program generally focuses on practicing abstinence from all substances (NAWS 2021). Importantly, NA has no structured costs for attendees, which makes the program one of, if not the most, cost-effective recovery program available to most people. Instead of membership fees, the program is self-supporting and reliant on members to offer the resources necessary for maintaining the program, which include people volunteering their time to host meetings and making monetary donations (Humphreys 2004, 1–31).

Like participating in other "mutual support" programs, participation in the NA program consists of attending meetings, completing readings, and engaging in peer sponsorship. The touchstone of the NA program is the local meetings, where NA members share their experiences and hear from peers who are practicing sobriety. Although meeting attendance is not required, NA recommends that people with substance use disorder attend "a meeting every day for at least 90 days to get to know NA members" and its program (NAWS 2024). The 12-step program references materials created by members in national NA leadership roles. The central resource for those attending NA meetings is the book *Narcotics Anonymous Basic Text*, which outlines the 12-step program and highlights narratives of recovery. Although the main text of the book has remained the same since its original publication in the 1980s, the book has been through revisions since then (White 2014, 13–20).

10.3.1 The NA 12-Step Program

NA outlines the 12-step program for recovery (see the left-hand side of Table 10.1). The first step states, "We admitted that we were powerless over our addiction, that our lives had become unmanageable." The steps continue with statements such as, "...a Power greater than ourselves could restore us to sanity," and "We humbly asked Him to remove our

Table 10.1 Comparisons of the 12-step items and CTR processes

12-step item	*CTR process(es) aligned*
1. We admitted that we were powerless over our addiction, that our lives had become unmanageable.	Foregrounding productive action while backgrounding negative feelings, putting alternative logics to work
2. We came to believe that a power greater than ourselves could restore us to sanity.	Affirming identity anchors, maintaining/using communication networks, putting alternative logics to work
3. We made a decision to turn our will and our lives over to the care of god as we understood him	Foregrounding productive action while backgrounding negative feelings, affirming identity anchors, maintaining/using communication networks
4. We made a searching and fearless moral inventory of ourselves.	Foregrounding productive action while backgrounding negative feelings
5. We admitted to god, to ourselves, and to another human being the exact nature of our wrongs.	Maintaining/using communication networks
6. We were entirely ready to have god remove all these defects of character.	Maintaining/using communication networks

(*continued*)

Table 10.1 (continued)

12-step item	*CTR process(es) aligned*
7. We humbly asked him to remove our shortcomings.	Foregrounding productive action while backgrounding negative feelings, maintaining/using communication networks
8. We made a list of all persons we had harmed, and became willing to make amends to them all.	Foregrounding productive action while backgrounding negative feelings, maintaining/using communication networks
9. We made direct amends to such people wherever possible, except when to do so would injure them or others.	Foregrounding productive action while backgrounding negative feelings, maintaining/using communication networks
10. We continued to take personal inventory and when we were wrong promptly admitted it.	Foregrounding productive action while backgrounding negative feelings, maintaining/using communication networks, putting alternative logics to work
11. We sought through prayer and meditation to improve our conscious contact with god as we understood him, praying only for knowledge of his will for us and the power to carry that out.	Crafting normalcy, foregrounding productive action while backgrounding negative feelings, maintaining/using communication networks
12. Having had a spiritual awakening as a result of these steps, we tried to carry this message to addicts, and to practice these principles in all our affairs.	Crafting normalcy, maintaining/using communication networks

Note. These items are printed in the *"Introductory Guide to Narcotics Anonymous"* (NAWS 2024). https://na.org/wp-content/uploads/2024/05/1200_Introductory-Guide-English.pdf

shortcomings" (NAWS 2024). The subsequent steps encourage individuals to seek support from a (nondenominational) higher power, make amends for previous transgressions, and commit to sobriety via self-improvement. Peer support is central to these steps. People with OUD benefit from the support of their peers in the NA group and are then expected to return the favor by helping others when they are ready to assist others with OUD. In other words, those in recovery are expected to give back to NA through the future assistance of others. Members following these steps are expected to be "living a clean life," meaning that they are not currently using any substances. Although, new attendees are welcome to attend even if they are "still using drugs, detoxing from drugs, or on drug replacement therapy" (NAWS 2024).

10.3.2 *Criticisms of the NA 12-Step Program*

Despite its widespread adoption around the world, the NA program is not without criticism. The central role of religion is one point of critique, as the program encourages reliance on a "higher power," which was previously specified as God. Although an increasing number of U.S. adults identify as being nonreligious (approximately 30%; Pew Research Center 2025), NA does not offer a secular recovery option. Additionally, some specialists argue that the strict emphasis on total abstinence by the NA program does not align with evidence-based harm-reduction models or medical treatment for OUD that uses medications such as methadone (Moos 2008, 387–96). Complete abstinence, although not required, restricts members from the use of approved medication for OUD. Even though the program would permit members using methadone to attend NA meetings, it considers the use of such medication, even when prescribed by a doctor, as points of relapse. This misconception has been criticized by medical organizations like the National Institutes of Health and by people with OUD who have attended NA meetings (Scherzer et al. 2022, 27; National Institute on Drug Abuse 2025). Researchers interviewing people with OUD who had attended NA meetings heard criticisms like, "Plus with AA and NA, I'm on Suboxone, so they don't consider me being clean. It's like what's the point of going?" (Scherzer et al. 2022, 27). Discouraging the use of medication such as buprenorphine and methadone is concerning given that treating OUD with these medications is the only proven method of reducing risk of overdose for people with OUD (Wakeman et al. 2020, 7).

The NA program also refers to all members as "addicts," which is an identity-label that is not resolved even after long-term recovery. The stigmatizing language used by the program is often in direct contrast to the recommendations of health professionals and communication researchers. Instead of using terms like "addict" and "staying clean," terms like "person with opioid use disorder" and "not currently using opioids" can be more inclusive and less likely to perpetuate stigma about OUD (Wolfe and Scharp 2022, 2936–2944). The use of stigmatizing terms was reflected by a person with OUD who attended NA meetings, "At least with me personally, the AA meetings and NA meetings. Those...made it worse for me, cuz listenin' to people's stories and talking about it and being around a lot of the other drug addicts, it made almost a community feel for me where I'm, 'Okay, well'—I mean, or it's okay to slip up" (Scharp et al. 2022, 28). Thus, for some people with OUD in the process of recovery, the stigmatizing terms may lead to internalized beliefs that they are just like their peers who are still using the substance, which is not helpful for recovery (Scharp et al. 2022, 27).

Moreover, researchers have called for more rigorous testing of the effectiveness of the NA program compared to other treatment methods. There is little data on the effectiveness of the NA program and peer recovery support services in general. In a meta-analysis examining peer recovery support services for OUD, including NA, the researchers were unable to make comparisons across any of the studies (Gormley et al. 2021, 109–123). The peer services offered were not standardized, the details of meetings were not tracked, the sample sizes were too small, and too many participants left the groups to make meaningful comparisons across interventions. Thus, rigorous research is needed to examine the effectiveness of these peer support services and how such programs might better address noted limitations.

10.4 Examining the NA 12-Step Program Via the CTR

A central critique of the 12-Step program is the lack of formative research about peer recovery mutual-support groups. Given our unique positions as communication researchers, we examined how the NA steps aligned with the communicative resilience processes proposed by the CTR. Given that the NA program is infrequently evaluated and researched for efficacy, the CTR can serve as a guideline for comparing the recommendations of the program to social scientific evidence about how to overcome adversity via communication (Scharp et al. 2021, 395–417; Wilson et al. 2021, 478–513; Scharp et al. 2022, 1–30; Geary et al. 2023, 91–108; Scharp et al. 2024, 345–360; Hintz et al. 2024, 2510–2523; Wolfe et al. 2024, 418–456). Table 1 includes the 12-step program as well as the corresponding CTR processes identified as aligning with each step.

In the remainder of this section, we discuss the process and the results of our analysis of the NA 12-step program via the lens of the CTR. When conducting the analysis, we first identified the six resilience-promoting processes outlined by the CTR and the 12-step program promoted by NA. We then met to discuss potential areas of overlap and divergence between the NA 12-step program and the CTR resilience-promoting processes. Our analysis identified five resilience processes that are encouraged by the program, with three of them overlapping with most phases of the 12-step program. Crafting normalcy and putting alternative logics to work align with a few of the 12 steps, and they were identified in the NA program less often than foregrounding productive action while backgrounding negative emotion, affirming identity anchors, and maintaining and using communication networks.

Foregrounding productive action while backgrounding negative feelings occurs when an individual emphasizes beneficial activities and discursively downplays negativity related to OUD (Buzzanell 2010, 1–14). This process was identified in a majority of the 12-step items, with statements such as "...admitted that we were powerless," "...made a decision to turn our will and lives over," and "...made a searching and fearless moral inventory of ourselves" (NAWS 2021). These statements center on the importance of action in recovery rather than dwelling on the emotions associated with OUD and recovery. The items also prompt members to make "direct amends" to others before seeking "prayer and meditation" for themselves (NAWS 2021). Thus, the 12-step program puts a priority on productive actions to become abstinent from substances, and then apologize to others, before engaging in activities to manage one's own emotions.

The other two CTR processes that align closely with the 12-step program are affirming identity anchors and maintaining and using communication networks. Affirming identity anchors occurs when an individual emphasizes their familial, community, or religious connections following OUD (Buzzanell 2010). Maintaining and using communication networks refers to people engaging with existing networks, reducing contact with unhelpful network connections, or forming new networks (Buzzanell 2019). These two CTR processes are somewhat combined in the 12-step program. Many items reference a "Power," "God," or "Him," which could be considered as an affirmation of a Christian identity and/or the maintenance or creation of a communication relationship with the referenced religious figurehead. The interpretation of these items could vary depending on whether this connection to a "higher power" is a new identity and relationship (i.e., a change toward religious identification) or a previously integrated aspect of their life (i.e., a continuation of an existing religious identity). Nevertheless, in addition to taking the steps recommended by the NA program, becoming an NA member is itself the enactment of affirming identity anchors and creating a new communication network.

Crafting normalcy is promoted when the NA program encourages people with OUD to create or return to routines. Individuals craft normalcy through actively creating new routines or maintaining an existing schedule. The last two items of the NA program promote the creation of normalcy by aiming to "improve our conscious contact with God" and "carry this message to addicts, and to practice these principles in all our affairs" (Buzzanell 2019, 65–88). In other words, these steps instruct members to formalize their interactions with "God" and establish these 12 steps as part of daily life. The NA program also facilitates crafting normalcy by suggesting that new members attend daily NA meetings for three months (NAWS 2024). This recommendation asks members to build a new daily schedule that allocates time for program meetings. This new schedule might also be required by court orders that mandate NA meeting attendance as a condition for release. Thus, the NA 12-step program (including its format) encourages the enactment of crafting normalcy among people with OUD.

Putting alternative logics to work is a resilience-promoting process that was also identified in several of the 12-step items alongside other CTR processes. This process occurs when people reframe their experience with a stressor via humor, metaphors, or novel ways of thinking about the situation (Hintz et al. 2021, 371–380). In the NA program, this process takes the form of positioning OUD as being beyond the control of the person (i.e., the notion that we are powerless over our OUD) and in the hands of "…a Power greater than ourselves" (NAWS 2021). This reframing is almost exclusively promoted in the initial steps of the 12-step program, which might help members begin with a preliminary reorientation to their OUD before engaging in other CTR processes. This push toward reframing also integrates affirming identity anchors by positioning OUD as being under the control of a (Christian) "higher power" with whom members develop or maintain a relationship.

We found that almost every phase of the 12-step program corresponded to more than one of the CTR resilience-promoting processes. This is notable given that building the resilience needed to respond to OUD likely requires multiple resources working together. Indeed, CTR research has found that people experiencing various trigger events rarely enact just one resilience-promoting process. For instance, people who experienced instances of identity-related discrimination found that the enactment of maintaining communication networks, foregrounding productive action, and putting alternative logics to work were helpful for building resilience with their face-to-face networks (Wolfe et al. 2024, 418–456). Moreover, combining crafting normalcy and putting alternative logics to work was found to build resilience productively (Scharp et al. 2024, 335–361). These findings can inform future recommendations to NA members and people with OUD about how to select resilience-promoting processes and combine multiple steps of the NA program to personalize their recovery process.

10.5 Discussion: Misalignment and Future Considerations

The preceding discussion of the NA 12-step program suggests that the program can be adjusted to better serve people battling substance use disorders, specifically OUD. Although affirming identity anchors through religiosity is prevalent across the 12-step program, the program does not explicitly encourage the affirmation of anchor identities beyond religious morality and adherence. As a large minority of U.S. adults are nonreligious (e.g., spiritual but not religious, agnostic, atheist; Pew Research Center 2025), the NA program could leverage the CTR to expand the range of identity anchors worth affirming in the search for recovery from OUD (Scharp et al. 2024, 335–361), such as those related to familial roles (e.g., being a "good" parent) or values unrelated to religiosity (e.g., honesty, gratitude, generosity). NA attendees' views of their religious identities may also influence how they engage with various phases of the 12-step program (e.g., what may comprise an alternative logic such as reframing). Some attendees may benefit from integrating their religious beliefs more fully in the program, whereas others may need to replace the reference to a "higher power" with a new touchpoint altogether. The NA program could adapt to the extent to which members affirm their identity anchors, depending on their comfortability as a step toward a personalized recovery and resilience plan. This would also allow NA to address the criticism that the organization currently does not offer a secular recovery option.

Maintaining and using communication networks could be discussed in terms of not only correcting past wrongdoings and establishing support from within NA, but also reducing contact with people who might encourage OUD or who have negative perceptions of treatment options using medication (Tsai et al. 2019). Utilizing communication networks could also include building a recovery team in addition to an NA network. NA facilitators are not medical or recovery experts. Instead, their expertise resides in shared life experiences with people who have used substances. NA peers do not need to be the only new network members that people integrate into their life following OUD. NA could encourage people to build a diverse group of peers and healthcare providers who can assist with the social and medical considerations of OUD. This recommendation could help decrease widespread negative perceptions of OUD and medical treatment for OUD (Hoffman et al. 2021, 108464).

The NA program could be augmented by further engagement with other resilience-promoting processes identified by the CTR. The NA program aligns with five of the CTR processes, with a strong engagement with three of the processes. There remain opportunities to better integrate the CTR processes into NA recommendations. For example, critiquing and resisting the status quo could be useful for addressing OUD. Specifically, the NA program could have their attendees identify environmental factors beyond their control (e.g., lack of economic opportunity) that contributed to their development of OUD and/or prevent them from seeking medical treatment for their disorder and make effort to mitigate those influences. These resistant efforts could include advocating for better public education programs about the dangers of opioids and mobilizing support for government funding of OUD recovery programs to increase the accessibility of such programs. Reducing the financial costs of recovery programs may allow people to choose the program that works best for them instead of selecting the NA program because it is free. Given the sociocultural complexities of OUD, acknowledging members' diverse identities, the necessity to prune existing OUD-related social networks, and addressing the societal factors that make OUD possible might further promote recovery and communicative resilience.

10.6 Conclusion

This chapter explores the extent to which the recommendations of the 12-step program promoted by Narcotics Anonymous (NA) map onto the six resilience-promoting processes outlined by the communication theory of resilience (CTR). Our analysis revealed that the NA 12-step program strongly encourages practices consistent with some CTR processes (e.g., foregrounding productive actions while backgrounding negative emotions) while largely failing to fully incorporate other CTR processes (e.g., critiquing the status quo). As enacting all six CTR processes has been illustrated to promote resilience over time when individuals are managing disruptive life events, our analysis suggests that the NA program could be further augmented by fully integrating otherwise-neglected CTR processes (Wilson et al. 2021, 478–513). In all, by identifying areas of overlap and opportunities for enhancement, we map the NA 12-step program onto the CTR to illuminate the potential empirical grounding of the program, as well as opportunities for improving the program through additional resilience practices.

References

Afifi, T. D. 2018. Individual/Relational Resilience. *Journal of Applied Communication Research* 46 (1): 5–9. https://doi.org/10.1080/00909882.2018.1426707.

Buzzanell, Patrice M. 2010. Resilience: Talking, Resisting, and Imagining New Normalcies into Being. *Journal of Communication* 60 (1): 1–14. https://doi.org/10.1111/j.1460-2466.2009.01469.x.

Buzzanell, Patrice M. 2018. Communication Theory of Resilience. In *Enacting Adaptive-Transformative Processes When Families Experience Loss and Disruption*, edited by Patrice M. Buzzanell. Routledge. https://doi.org/10.4324/9781315204321-9.

Buzzanell, Patrice M. 2019. Communication Theory of Resilience in Everyday Talk, Interactions, and Network Structures. In *Reflections on Interpersonal Communication Research*, edited by Steven R. Wilson and Sandy Smith. Cognella.

Buzzanell, Patrice M., and Lynn H. Turner. 2003. Emotion Work Revealed by Job Loss Discourse: Backgrounding-Foregrounding of Feelings, Construction of Normalcy, and (Re)Instituting of Traditional Masculinities. *Journal of Applied Communication Research* 31 (1): 27–57. https://doi.org/10.1080/00909880305375.

Geary, Devon, Kristina Scharp, and Valerie Manusov. 2023. Life Interrupted Instead of Disrupted: Triggers and Resilient Communication Processes Revealed in POZ.com Online Narratives by Men with HIV Who Have Sex with Men. *Journal of Applied Communication Research* 51 (1): 91–108. https://doi.org/10.1080/00909882.2022.2099227.

Gormley, Mirinda Ann, Irene Pericot-Valverde, Liam Diaz, et al. 2021. Effectiveness of Peer Recovery Support Services on Stages of the Opioid Use

Disorder Treatment Cascade: A Systematic Review. *Drugs and Alcohol Dependence* 229 (B): 109123. https://doi.org/10.1016/j.cct.2023.107235.

Harrison, Elizabeth. 2013. Bouncing Back? Recession, Resilience and Everyday Lives. *Critical Social Policy* 33 (1): 97–113. https://doi.org/10.1177/0261018312439365.

Hintz, Elizabeth A., Timothy Betts, and Patrice M. Buzzanell. 2021. Caring for Patients without Personal Protective Equipment (PPE): Material Conditions as Multidimensional Cascading Triggers for Resilience Processes. *Health Communication* 38 (2): 371–380. https://doi.org/10.1080/10410236.2021.1953727.

Hintz, Elizabeth A., Rachel V. Tucker, and Steve R. Wilson. 2024. Developing Measures for and Testing the Theory of Communicative Disenfranchisement (TCD) in the Context of Chronic Pain. *Health Communication* 39 (12): 2510–2523. https://doi.org/10.1080/10410236.2023.2275916.

Hoffman, Lauren A., Connie L. Vilsaint, and John F. Kelly. 2021. Attitudes Toward Opioid Use Disorder Pharmacotherapy Among Recovery Community Center Attendees. *Journal of Substance Abuse Treatment* 131:108464. https://doi.org/10.1016/j.jsat.2021.108464.

Humphreys, Keith. 2004. *Circles of Recovery: Self-Help Organizations for Addictions.* Cambridge University Press.

Moos, Rudolf H. 2008. Active Ingredients of Substance Use-Focused Self-Help Groups. *Addiction* 103 (3): 387–396.

Narcotics Anonymous World Services. 2024. Introduction to NA Meetings. https://na.org/wp-content/uploads/2024/05/EN3129-IP-29-English.pdf.

Narcotics Anonymous World Services. 2025. *Narcotics Anonymous.* https://na.org. Accessed 31 March 2025.

National Institute on Drug Abuse. 2025. *Words Matter – Terms to Use and Avoid When Talking About Addiction.* March 31. https://nida.nih.gov/nidamed-medical-health-professionals/health-professions-education/words-matter-terms-to-use-avoid-when-talking-about-addiction.

Pew Research Center. 2025. *Decline of Christianity in the U.S. Has Slowed, May Have Leveled Off.* February 26. https://www.pewresearch.org/religion/2025/02/26/decline-of-christianity-in-the-us-has-slowed-may-have-leveled-off/.

Scharp, Kristina M., Devon Geary, Brooke H. Wolfe, et al. 2021. Understanding the Triggers and Communication Processes That Constitute Resilience in the Context of Migration to the United States. *Communication Monographs* 88 (4): 395–417. https://doi.org/10.1080/03637751.2020.1856395.

Scharp, Kristina M., Tiffany R. Wang, and Brooke H. Wolfe. 2022. Communicative Resilience of First-Generation College Students During the COVID-19 Pandemic. *Human Communication Research* 48 (1): 1–30. https://doi.org/10.1093/hcr/hqab018.

Scharp, Kristina M., Cimmiaron F. Alvarez, Brooke H. Wolfe, et al. 2024. Overcoming Obstacles by Enacting Resilience: How Queer Adolescents Respond to Being Estranged from Their Parents. *Communication Research* 51 (3): 335–361. https://doi.org/10.1177/00936502221142175.

Scherzer, Caroline, Paulo Jiménez Muñoz, Susan Ramsey, et al. 2022. Perceptions of Medications, Program Settings, and Drug Use Histories Among Individuals Engaged in Treatment for Opioid Use Disorder. *Journal of Addictive Diseases* 42 (1): 24–32. https://doi.org/10.1080/10550887.2022.2126273.

Siegenthaler, Bianca, Jared V. Worwood, and Willow Craine. 2024. Patterns of Disruptions: Complexities of Discursive-Embodied Triggers and Resilience Responses of Individuals with Autoimmune Diseases. *Communication Monographs* 91 (3): 396–417. https://doi.org/10.1080/03637751.2023.2295461.

Tsai, Alexander C., Mathew V. Kiang, Barnett L. Beletsky, et al. 2019. Stigma as a Fundamental Hindrance to the United States Opioid Overdose Crisis Response. *PLoS Med* 16 (11): e1002969. https://doi.org/10.1371/journal.pmed.1002969.

Wakeman, Sarah E., Marc R. Larochelle, Omid Ameli, et al. 2020. Comparative Effectiveness of Different Treatment Pathways for Opioid Use Disorder. *JAMA Network Open* 3 (2): e1920622. https://doi.org/10.1001/jamanetworkopen.2019.20622.

White, William L. 2014. *Slaying the Dragon: The History of Addiction Treatment and Recovery in America*. Chestnut Health Systems.

Wilson, Steven R., Kai Kuang, Elizabeth A. Hintz, et al. 2021. Developing and Validating the Communication Resilience Process Scale. *Journal of Communication* 71 (3): 478–513. https://doi.org/10.1093/joc/jqab013.

Wolfe, Brooke H., and Kristina M. Scharp. 2022. A (In)curable Disease? Making Meaning of Addiction from the Perspective of People in Recovery from Opioid Use Disorder. *Health Communication* 38 (13): 2936–2944. https://doi.org/10.1080/10410236.2022.2128157.

Wolfe, Brooke H., Valerie Manusov, and Kristina M. Scharp. 2024. Building Resilience in Response to Identity-Based Discrimination through In Person and Online Communication. *Communication Monographs* 91 (3): 418–456. https://doi.org/10.1080/03637751.2023.2300821.

Index

X. Cao (ed.), *Fighting the Opioid Crisis with Communication*,
https://doi.org/10.1007/978-3-032-31162-7

FSC
www.fsc.org
MIX
Papier | Fördert
gute Waldnutzung
FSC® C083411

Kolibri 360 GmbH
Ferdinand-Jühlke-Straße 7
99095 Erfurt, Deutschland
produktsicherheit@kolibri360.de